PUBLIC HEALTH: PRACTICES, METHODS AND POLICIES

NIGERIA

PERSPECTIVES OF HEALTH

PUBLIC HEALTH: PRACTICES, METHODS AND POLICIES

JOAV MERRICK - SERIES EDITOR

MEDICAL DIRECTOR, HEALTH SERVICES, DIVISION FOR INTELLECTUAL AND DEVELOPMENTAL DISABILITIES, MINISTRY OF SOCIAL AFFAIRS AND SOCIAL SERVICES, JERUSALEM, ISRAEL

Nigeria: Perspectives of Health
Ariel Tenenbaum, Kehinde K Kanmod and Joav Merrick
(Editors)
2020. ISBN: 978-1-53618-090-9
(Softcover)
2020. ISBN: 978-1-53618-091-6
(e-book)

The COVID-19 Pandemic: A Tribute to the Corona Whistleblowers
Joav Merrick, Søren Ventegodt and Niels Jørgen Andersen
(Authors)
2020. ISBN: 978-1-53618-146-3
(Hardcover)
2020 ISBN: 978-1-53618-236-1
(e-book)

Advances in Chinese Children, Adolescent and Family Research
Ariel Tenenbaum, Daniel T.L. Shek, Moon YM Law and Joav Merrick
(Editors)
2020. ISBN: 978-1-53617-870-8
(Hardcover)
2020. ISBN. 978-1-53617-871-5
(e-book)

Child Environmental Health Disparities: Looking at the Present and Facing the Future
I. Leslie Rubin and Joav Merrick
(Editors)
2020. ISBN: 978-1-53617-823-4
(Hardcover)
2020. ISBN. 978-1-53617-824-1
(e-book)

Positive Youth Development: Digital Game-Based Learning
Ty Lee, Daniel T.L. Shek, Sarah Sw Lee, and Joav Merrick (Editors)
2020. ISBN: 978-1-53617-795-4 (Hardcover)
2020. ISBN. 978-1-53617-796-1 (e-book)

Service Leadership Education in an Era of Service Economy
Daniel TL Shek, Xiaoqin Zhu, and Joav Merrick (Editors)
2020. ISBN: 978-1-53617-514-1 (Hardcover)
2020. ISBN: 978-1-53617-515-8 (e-book)

Parenting and Family Life in a Chinese Society
Daniel TL Shek, Moon YM Law, Joav Merrick (Editors)
2020. ISBN: 978-1-53616-705-4 (Softcover)
2020. ISBN: 978-1-53616-706-1 (e-book)

Public Health: Topics, Themes and Trends
Satesh Bidaisee, Sadik Uddin Emmanuel Keku, Joav Merrick (Editors)
2020. ISBN: 978-1-53616-655-2 (Softcover)
2020. ISBN: 978-1-53616-656-9

Public Health: Environment and Child Health in a Changing World
I. Leslie Rubin and Joav Merrick (Editors)
2019. ISBN: 978-1-53615-394-1 (Hardcover)
2019. ISBN: 978-1-53615395-8 (e-book)

Service Leadership: Tools to Assess Knowledge, Attitude and Behavior
Daniel TL Shek, Xiaoqin Zhu, Li Lin and Joav Merrick (Editors)
2019. ISBN: 978-1-53614-852-7 (Hardcover)
2019. ISBN: 978-1-53614-853-4 (e-book)

Public Health Yearbook 2017
Joav Merrick (Editor)
2018. ISBN: 978-1-53613-792-7 (Hardcover)
2018. ISBN: 978-1-53613-793-4 (e-book)

Resilience and Health: A Potent Dynamic
I Leslie Rubin and Joav Merrick (Editors)
2018. ISBN: 978-1-53613-412-4 (Hardcover)
2018. ISBN: 978-1-53613-413-1 (e-book)

Medical History: Some Perspectives Second Edition
Donald E. Greydanus and Joav Merrick, (Editors)
2018. ISBN: 978-1-53613-319-6 (Hardcover)
2018. ISBN: 978-1-53613-320-2 (e-book)

University Students: Promotion of Holistic Development in Hong Kong
Daniel TL Shek, Lu Yu and Joav Merrick (Editors)
2017. ISBN: 978-1-53612-535-1 (Hardcover)
2017. ISBN: 978-1-53612-537-5 (e-book)

Alzheimer's Disease: Awareness among Young Adults
Ronald Chow, Drew Hollenberg, Michael Borean and Joav Merrick (Editors)
2017. ISBN: 978-1-53612-456-9 (Softcover)
2017. ISBN: 978-1-53612-457-6 (e-book)

Service Leadership Education for University Students
Daniel TL Shek, Po Chung, Li Lin and Joav Merrick (Editors)
2017. ISBN: 978-1-53611-949-7 (Hardcover)
2017. ISBN: 978-1-53611-969-5 (e-book)

Leadership: Promoting Leadership and Intrapersonal Development in University Students
Daniel TL Shek, Cecilia MS Ma and Joav Merrick (Editors)
2017. ISBN: 978-1-53611-950-3 (Hardcover)
2017. ISBN: 978-1-53611-970-1 (e-book)

Caribbean Adolescents: Misuse and Abuse of Alcohol
Cecilia Hegamin-Younger and Joav Merrick (Editors)
2017. ISBN: 978-1-63485-880-9 (Hardcover)
2016. ISBN: 978-1-63485-894-6 (e-book)

Public Health: An Ecological Framework for Child Environmental Health Interventions
I. Leslie Rubin and Joav Merrick (Editors)
2017. ISBN: 978-1-53610-700-5 (Hardcover)
2017. ISBN: 978-1-53610-714-2 (e-book)

Diabetes Mellitus: A Medical History Journey
Donald E. Greydanus and Joav Merrick
2016. ISBN: 978-1-53610-094-5 (Softcover)
2016. ISBN: 978-1-53610-103-4 (e-book)

Education in Hong Kong: Service Leadership for University Students
Daniel TL Shek, Cecilia MS Ma, Li Lin and Joav Merrick (Editors)
2016. ISBN: 978-1-63484-928-9 (Hardcover)
2016. ISBN: 978-1-63484-960-9 (e-book)

Environmental Health Disparities: Costs and Benefits of Breaking the Cycle
I. Leslie Rubin and Joav Merrick (Editors)
2016. ISBN: 978-1-63484-211-2 (Hardcover)
2016. ISBN: 978-1-63484-212-9 (e-book)

Higher Education in Hong Kong: Nurturing Students to be Caring Service Leaders
Daniel TL Shek, Andrew MH Siu, Hildie Leung and Joav Merrick (Editors)
2016. ISBN: 978-1-63484-980-7 (Hardcover)
2016. ISBN: 978-1-63485-009-4 (e-book)

Measles: Epidemiology and Control of Measles in the Gweru Urban District in Zimbabwe
Tawanda Marufu, Seter Siziya, Mazyanga L. Mazaba and Joav Merrick (Editors)
2016. ISBN: 978-1-63485-559-4 (Hardcover)
2016. ISBN: 978-1-63485-573-0 (e-book)

Medical History: Some Perspectives
Donald E. Greydanus and Joav Merrick
2016. ISBN: 978-1-63484-747-6 (Hardcover)
2016. ISBN: 978-1-63484-849-7 (e-book)

Public Health: Some International Aspects
Joav Merrick (Editor)
2016. ISBN: 978-1-63484-612-7 (Hardcover)
2016. ISBN: 978-1-63484-630-1 (e-book)

Public Health: International Aspects on Environment and Health
I. Leslie Rubin and Joav Merrick (Editors)
2016. ISBN: 978-1-63484-834-3 (Hardcover)
2016. ISBN: 978-1-63484-849-7 (e-book)

Smoking and Adolescence: International Public Health Experiences
Mazyanga L. Mazaba, Seter Siziya and Joav Merrick (Editors)
2016. ISBN: 978-1-63484-311-9 (Hardcover)
2016. ISBN: 978-1-63484-312-6 (e-book)

Arbovirus: Public Health Experience from Zambia
Seter Siziya, Mazyanga L. Mazaba, and Joav Merrick (Editors)
2015. ISBN: 978-1-63463-601-8 (Hardcover)
2015. ISBN: 978-1-63463-618-6 (e-book)

Health Issues in Diverse Cultures
Cecilia Obeng, Samuel Gyasi Obeng and Joav Merrick (Editors)
2015. ISBN: 978-1-63463-613-1 (Hardcover)
2015. ISBN: 978-1-63463-619-3 (e-book)

Public Health, Social Work and Health Inequalities
Bruce D. Friedman and Joav Merrick (Editors)
2015. ISBN: 978-1-63482-838-3 (Hardcover)
2015. ISBN: 978-1-63482-850-5 (e-book)

Patient Dumping: Background, Protections, and the Mentally Ill
Tabitha E. Rivers (Editor)
2015. ISBN: 978-1-63483-726-2 (Hardcover)
2015. ISBN: 978-1-63483-727-9 (e-book)

Tomorrow's Leaders: Service Leadership and Holistic Development in Chinese University Students
Daniel TL Shek, Andrew MH Siu and Joav Merrick (Editors)
2015. ISBN: 978-1-63321-880-2 (Hardcover)
2014. ISBN: 978-1-63321-943-4 (e-book)

Environment and Public Health: Environmental Health, Law and International Perspectives
I. Leslie Rubin and Joav Merrick (Editors)
2014. ISBN: 978-1-63463-167-9 (Hardcover)
2014. ISBN: 978-1-63463-189-1 (e-book)

PUBLIC HEALTH: PRACTICES, METHODS AND POLICIES

NIGERIA

PERSPECTIVES OF HEALTH

ARIEL TENENBAUM
KEHINDE K. KANMODI
AND
JOAV MERRICK
EDITORS

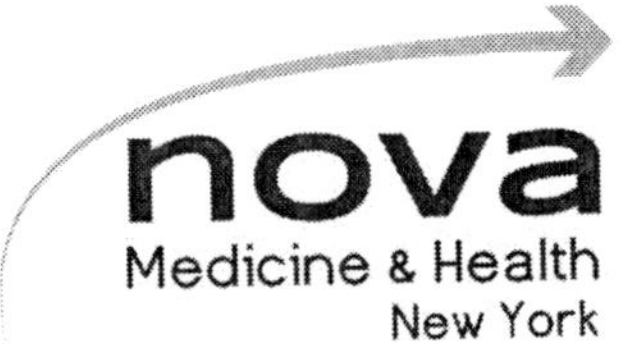

Library of Congress Cataloging-in-Publication Data

Names: Tenenbaum, Ariel, editor. | Kanmodi, Kehinde K., editor. | Merrick, Joav, 1950- editor.
Title: Nigeria: perspectives of health / [edited by] Kehinde Kazeem Kanmodi, BDS, Cephas Health Research Initiative Inc, Ibadan, Nigeria,
Mental and Oral Health Development Organization, Birnin Kebbi, Nigeria, Department of Community Health, Aminu Musa Habib College of Health Science and Techology, Yauri, Nigeria, Ariel Tenenbaum, MD, Center for Children with Chronic Diseases and Down Syndrome Center Jerusalem, Israel, and Joav Merrick, MD, MMedSci, DMSc, Department of Pediatrics, Mt Scopus Campus, Hadassah Hebrew University Medical Center, Jerusalem, Israel, National Institute of Child Health and Human Development, Jerusalem, Israel, Kentucky Children's Hospital, University of Kentucky, Lexington, Kentucky, United States and Center for Healthy Development, School of Public Health, Georgia State University, Atlanta, United States of America.
Identifiers: LCCN 2020024379 (print) | LCCN 2020024380 (ebook) | ISBN 9781536180909 (paperback) | ISBN 9781536180916 (adobe pdf)
Subjects: LCSH: Traditional medicine--Nigeria. | Medical care--Nigeria. | Social medicine--Nigeria. | Nigeria--Social life and customs.
Classification: LCC RA418.3.N6 N53 2020 (print) | LCC RA418.3.N6 (ebook) | DDC 362.109669--dc23
LC record available at https://lccn.loc.gov/2020024379
LC ebook record available at https://lccn.loc.gov/2020024380

Published by Nova Science Publishers, Inc. † New York

CONTENTS

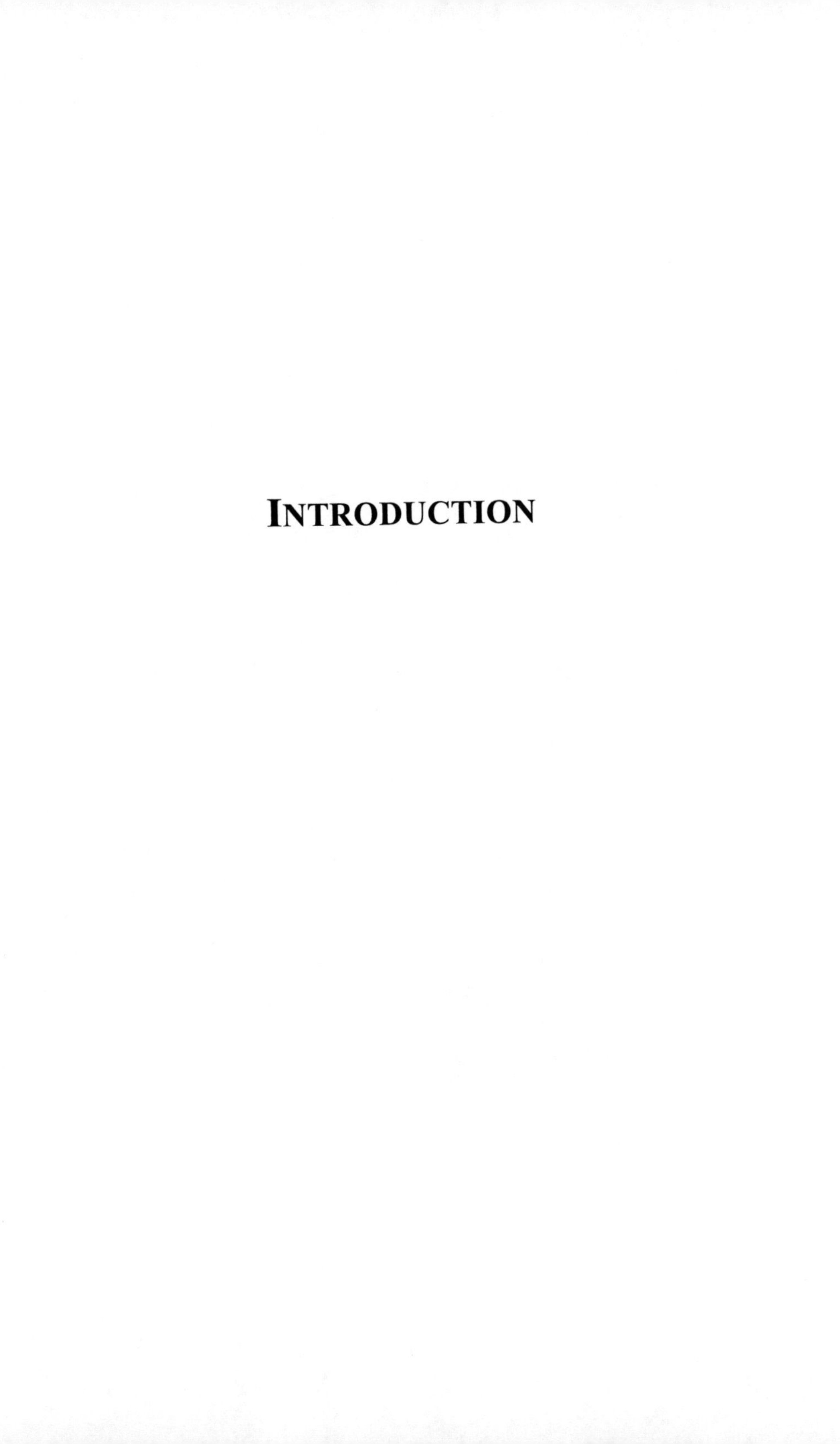

INTRODUCTION

In: Nigeria: Perspectives of Health
Editors: Ariel Tenenbaum et al.
ISBN: 978-1-53618-090-9

Chapter 1

HEALTH AND THE NIGERIAN SOCIETY: AN OVERVIEW

Kehinde K. Kanmodi[1-3,*], BDS,
Ariel Tenenbaum[4], MD
and Joav Merrick[5-8], MD, MMedSci, DMSc

[1]Cephas Health Research Initiative Inc, Ibadan, Nigeria, [2]Mental and Oral Health Development Organization, Birnin Kebbi, Nigeria, [3]Department of Community Health, Aminu Musa Habib College of Health Science and Techology, Yauri, Nigeria, [4]Center for Children with Chronic Diseases and Down Syndrome Center Jerusalem, Israel, [5]Department of Pediatrics, Mt Scopus Campus, Hadassah Hebrew University Medical Center, Jerusalem, Israel, [6]National Institute of Child Health and Human Development, Jerusalem, Israel, [7]Kentucky Children's Hospital, University of Kentucky, Lexington, Kentucky, United States of America and [8]Center for Healthy Development, School of Public Health, Georgia State University, Atlanta, Georgia, United States of America

[*] Corresponding Author's Email: kehindekanmodi@gmail.com.

ABSTRACT

Nigeria – a pluralistic society – is a sub-Saharan Africa country, home to about 200 million people from 371 cultural tribes. All tribes in Nigeria have their specific cultural beliefs and practices. As a matter of fact, many of these practices had been in existence for hundreds of years, even before British colonization (1800-1960). There exists a strong interrelationship between the society and health. Some practices in the society have negative health implications while some do not. Unfortunately, many of the traditional or cultural practices in the Nigerian society have more associated harms than benefits. In this book we have gathered research that describes health and health aspects of modern Nigeria, which we hope will be of interest to the reader.

INTRODUCTION

It is a popular saying that health is wealth. This statement is actually true. The health of a person goes far a long way in determining their wealth. Similarly, a healthy society is a wealthy society.

A society, according to the Cambridge dictionary is “a large group of people who live together in an organized way, making decisions about how to do things and sharing the work that needs to be done” (1). All the people in a country, or in several similar countries, can be referred to as a society (1).

NIGERIAN SOCIETY

There are 36 states in Nigeria, excluding the Federal Capital Territory (FCT) which is situated in Abuja (see figure 1) (2). These 36 states spread across the wix geopolitical zones of the country (see Table 1). The Nigerian political system is democracy, adopting the United States presidential structure of governance (3).

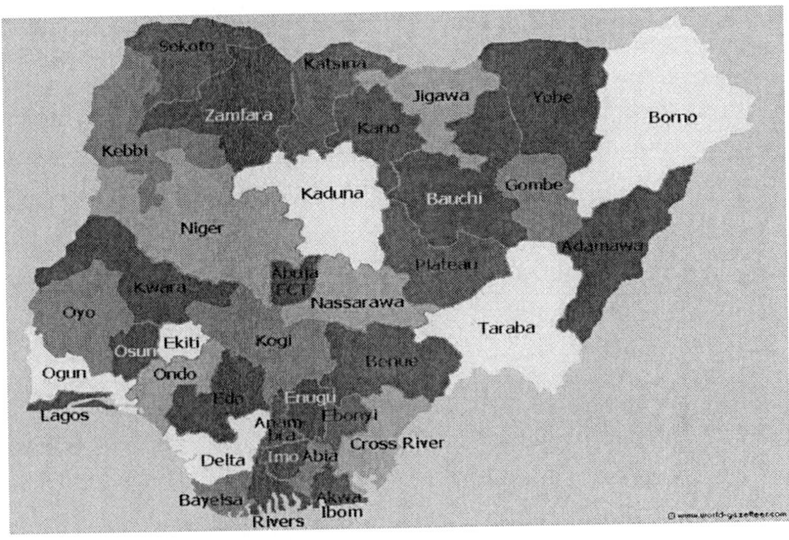

Figure 1. Map of Nigeria showing all the 36 states with the federal capital territory.

Table 1. Geopolitical zones of Nigeria

Geopolitical zone	State
South-west	Osun, Oyo, Ondo, Ogun, Ekiti, Lagos
South-east	Abia, Anambra, Ebonyi, Enugu, Imo
South-south	Akwa Ibom, Bayelsa, Cross River, Edo, Delta, Rivers
North-central	Benue, Kogi, Nasarawa, Plateau, Niger, Kwara, Federal Capital Territory
North-east	Borno, Bauchi, Gombe, Taraba, Yobe, Adamawa
North-west	Sokoto, Kebbi, Zamfara, Katsina, Kaduna, Jigawa, Kano

Nigeria – a pluralistic society – is a sub-Saharan Africa country, home to about 200 million people from 371 cultural tribes (4, 5). Amongst all the cultural tribes in Nigeria, Yoruba, Hausa/Fulani and Igbo are the three major tribes (5). The northern part of Nigeria is predominantly occupied by the Hausa/Fulani ethnic group while the southern part of Nigeria is predominantly occupied by the Yoruba and the Igbo ethnic groups (5).

Cultural beliefs and practices in Nigeria

All tribes in Nigeria have their specific cultural beliefs and practices. As a matter of fact, many of these practices had been in existence for hundreds of years, even before British colonization (1800-1960) (6). Health-wise, some beliefs and practices are favorable, while some are not (6, 7). In this chapter, we shall briefly mention some popular cultural beliefs and practices and their health implications in the Nigerian society (see Table 2).

Table 2. Examples of popular cultural beliefs and practices in Nigeria

Part of Nigeria	Beliefs/practice	Purpose/understanding	Health implication
Northern	Sakkiya	To cure body swelling	Negative; controversial
Northern	Kawo	To cure body swelling	Negative; controversial
Northern	Kamun wuta	To cure severe burns	Negative; controversial
Northern	Dauri	To treat limb fracture	Negative; controversial
Southern	Te Magun	To punish women who are not faithful in their marriage	Negative
Southern	Eji beauty	Epitome of feminine beauty	Nil`

In the Hausa culture, for instance, there is a popular traditional practice called Sakkiya (8). Sakkiya is an act of using a hot pointed metallic tip to puncture a body swelling with the hope of achieving a curative effect (8). This procedure is widely practiced in rural villages in northern Nigeria commonly by the blacksmith (called Makera) and traditional barbers (called wanzami) (9). Scientific investigations has shown that this traditional practice can be lethal due to its queried safety profile and associated complications that may arise from it (7, 10). Also, there exist some other traditional practices in this region such as Kawo, Kamun wuta,

Dauri, etc. The Kawo practice involves the use of the human mouth to suck out the fluid content in a body swelling via horn of a ram (the horn of the ram serves as a straw to suck the fluid). Kamun wuta is a spiritual procedure that involves the use of special ritual and the application of locally prepared special powder on severe burns; this procedure is being done by Malams (spiritualists), it is not hygienic and it is done with the purpose of curing burns. Dauri is known as traditional bone setting and it involves the use of sticks and bandages to support fractured limbs. Dauri is being done by Malams. These cultural practices towards are crude and harmful to human health.

In the Yoruba culture, there is a popular practice called "te Magun" ("te" means placing while Magun refers to "thunderbolt"). This practice the placing of magical thread on door threshold for a woman to inadvertently walk over it and be under the spell; if any woman walks over it and she fails to have penetrative vaginal intercourse with any man within seven days after, she will emaciate and dry; however, if she does, the man will die after the intercourse. For the men that fell victim of such, they may crow or somersault three times, and die immediately. The "te Magun" is used in the Yoruba culture to punish married women who are not faithful to their spouse. Also, there is a belief that midline diastema (called "Eji" in Yoruba language) is a mark of epitome of beauty. Women with "Eji" are more appealing to the men in the Yoruba society than those without "Eji". Due to this societal perception on "Eji", some women do patronize quacks who are parading themselves as dentist to have a gap created in-between their upper central incisors. In the course of getting a gap tooth, some women sustain/develop dental traumas and/or odontogenic infections.

In the Igbo culture, the midline diastema ("Eji" belief in Yoruba culture) is also believed to be a mark of magnificent beauty among Igbo women. Some Igbo women do seek quacks for gap creation in between their teeth; unfortunately, this practice has negative oral health implications (such as tooth fracture, dentinal hypersensitivity) that can be incurred.

Conclusion

There exists a strong interrelationship between the society and health. Some practices in the society have negative health implications while some do not. Unfortunately, many of the traditional or cultural practices in the Nigerian society have more associated harms than benefits.

References

[1] Cambridge Dictionary (Online). Society. URL: https://dictionary.cambridge.org/dictionary/english/society.

[2] NigeriaGalleria. Nigerian 36 states and capital, governors. URL: https://www.nigeriagalleria.com/Nigeria/Nigerian-States-Capital-Governors.html.

[3] Brown GM. Nigerian political system: An analysis. Int J Human Soc Sci 2013;3(10):172-9.

[4] World Bank. Population, total – Nigeria. URL: https://data.worldbank.org/indicator/SP.POP.TOTL?locations=NG.

[5] Vanguard. List of all 371 tribes in Nigeria, states where they originate. URL: https://www.vanguardngr.com/2017/05/full-list-of-all-371-tribes-in-nigeria-states-where-they-originate/.

[6] Kanmodi KK, Almu B, Sani S, Ibrahim S, Owadokun AM, Adeniyi OR, et al. Sakkiya training and practice: A brief research report. J Altern Med Res 2018;10(4):363-7.

[7] Kanmodi K, Ndubuizu G, Owoeye O. Cause for concern on the negative health implications of the traditional Sakkiya treatment: Evidence from a survey of clinicians domiciled in a northern Nigerian academic hospital. J Altern Med Res 2018;10(4):349-54.

[8] Kanmodi KK. Sakkiya treatment in northern Nigeria: Any existing scientific literature? J Altern Med Res 2018;10(4):311-3.

[9] Kanmodi KK, Owoeye OI, Ndubuizu GO. Caregiver reports on the socio-economic and safety issues associated with Sakkiya treatment: a survey of a neglected area in Nigerian healthcare. Int Public Health J 2018;10(2):197-203.

[10] Kanmodi KK, Almu B, Sani S, Ibrahim S. The Sakkiya doctor and the Sakkiya clinic: Findings from a field work. J Altern Med Res 2018;10(4):355-61.

[11] Alabi EM. Cultural practices in Nigeria. Newsl Inter Afr Comm Tradit Pract Affect Health Women Child 1990;(9):6-7.

SECTION ONE: HEALTH ASPECTS

In: Nigeria: Perspectives of Health
Editors: Ariel Tenenbaum et al.
ISBN: 978-1-53618-090-9

Chapter 2

OPINIONS OF NIGERIAN RELIGIOUS LEADERS AND SEMINARIANS ON WHAT CAUSES CANCER

Adewale I Badru[1], MBBS, FMCA,
Kehinde K Kanmodi[2,*], BDS, Dip FM, PGDPM, PDGE, PGDPSCR, CPMP, ACIPM,
Precious A Ogundipe[1,3], BSc, MSc,
Andrew M Owadokun[2,4], MBBS
and Miracle A Adesina[2], BPT

[1]Emergency Department, University College Hospital, Ibadan
[2]Cephas Health Research Initiative Inc, Ibadan
[3]Department of Statistics, Federal University of Technology, Akure
[4]International Bible Training College, Port Harcourt, Nigeria

* Corresponding Author's Email: kanmodikehinde@yahoo.com.

Abstract

Many cancer patients in Nigeria present very late at hospitals for treatment. Studies have shown that the delay is due to the belief that their cancer disease is of a spiritual cause. In this chapter we explore the opinions of religious leaders and seminarians in Ibadan City, Oyo State, Nigeria, on the top five aetiology/risk factors of cancer. Methods: A cross-sectional study was done among 302 religious leaders and seminarians in Ibadan. Study tool was an anonymous questionnaire. Data collected was analysed using SPSS version 16 software. Results: The top five cancer aetiology/risk factors, as indicated by the respondents, were as follows: toxic drugs (58.9%); genetic factors (53.6%); radiation exposure (52%); poison (42.4%); poverty (34.8%). Conclusion: The opinion of the majority of the surveyed religious leaders and seminarians favoured biological, physical and chemical factors as the commonest cancer aetiology/risk factors, although the minority were of the opinion that cancer can also be caused by socioeconomic factors and supernatural forces.

Introduction

The prevalence of cancer disease is on the increase among Nigerians, and also among the inhabitants of other developing nations (1, 2). As far back as 2008, about 12.7 million cancer cases and 7.6 million cancer deaths have been reported worldwide, of which 56% of these cases and 64% of these deaths occurred in the developing countries, Nigeria inclusive (3).

It is so unfortunate that many cancer patients in Nigeria do delay their presentation at hospitals, unlike those in the developed world (4-8). Many of these patients do present at the hospital when their cancer disease is already at its advanced stage (4, 6-8). As a matter of fact, one of the main reasons for their delay in seeking hospital care is that many of them ascribed their cancer disease to spiritual causes (4, 6, 7) and many of these patients had first sought spiritual healing by visiting prayer houses, traditional healers, and spiritualists, before eventually presenting at the hospital after their attempts towards achieving spiritual healing of the cancer disease proofed abortive (4-6).

In Nigeria, the religious leaders have a strong influence on their followers. In many cases, they are being referred to as someone next to God. At times, people consult them for healing prayers, blessings, and counselling. Similarly, the seminarians who are the future religious leaders, usually occupy leadership positions in the religious institutions where they find themselves. The seminarians are also, though to a lesser extent, consulted for prayers and counselling too.

Since the religious leaders and seminarians are visited for healing prayers, it will be of importance to conduct a study to explore their opinions on the common risk factors of cancer, as the information obtained will determine their level of awareness on the evidence-based cancer aetiology and risk factors. Based on the above, we aim to write a short report on the opinions of a sample of religious leaders and seminarians in Ibadan City, Nigeria, on the most common causes of cancer in the Nigerian society.

OUR STUDY

This study was a descriptive cross-sectional study. This study also forms part of a bigger study conducted among religious leaders and seminarians in Ibadan, Nigeria (9), which adopted the use of same methodology.

However, the study tool used in this present study was a paper semi-structured questionnaire which obtained information on the socio-demographic characteristics of the participants, and the five commonest causes of cancer in the Nigerian society.

A total of 350 participants were recruited for this study. Each of the participants was given a questionnaire to fill and return. After the retrieval of the administered questionnaires, only 311 questionnaires were found filled. Out of the 311 filled questionnaires, only 9 were discarded because they were not filled properly, so we finally worked on the data from 302 respondents. Research data were entered into the SPSS version 16 software for analysis. The frequency distributions of all variables were determined, and test of association between two non-continuous variables were done using the Chi-square test. A significant p-value was recorded as <0.05.

This study was conducted under strict compliance with the 1964 Helsinki Declaration on health research involving human subjects.

FINDINGS

The demographic characteristics of the respondents had been presented earlier in a paper by Badru and Kanmodi (9). Table 1 depicts the opinions of the respondents on the causes of cancer in the Nigerian society. The top five cancer aetiology/risk factors, as indicated by the respondents, are as follows: toxic drugs (58.9%); genetic factors (53.6%); radiation exposure (52%); poison (42.4%) and poverty (34.8%).

Table 1. Association between gender of respondents and their opinion on the commonest cancer causes

Cancer causes	**Frequency (%) [N = 302]**
Sin	79 (26.2)
Evil spirit	85 (28.1)
God	17 (5.6)
Radiation exposure	157 (52.0)
Toxic drugs	178 (58.9)
Genetic factor	162 (53.6)
Generational curses	66 (21.9)
Witchcraft	58 (19.2)
Poison	128 (42.4)
Wealth	57 (18.9)
Poverty	105 (34.8)

DISCUSSION

The Nigerian religious leaders are known to have strong influence over their followers; these leaders bear different religious titles such as Pastor, Reverend, Evangelist, Imam, Alfas, among others. The pastors, evangelists, reverends, and missionaries are of the Christian faith, while the Imams and Alfas are of the Islamic faith. These religious leaders see to the social and spiritual welfare of their followers. On many occasions, they organize sessions of healing prayers for their sick followers. The seminarians, on the other hand, are trainees hoping to become a religious leader someday. As a matter of fact, some seminarians are likewise actively engaged in religious leadership positions in the Nigerian society.

This study was conducted to explore the opinions of religious leaders and seminarians in the metropolitan city of Ibadan, Nigeria, on the five most common causes of cancer in the Nigerian society. The findings made from this study revealed diverse opinions on this issue of concern, and these opinions are noteworthy. It is interesting to note that roughly one-quarter believed that sin can cause cancer disease. The Merriam-Webster Dictionary defines sin as: an offense against religious or moral law; an action that is or is felt to be highly reprehensible; an often serious shortcoming; a transgression of the law of God; or a vitiated state of human nature in which the self is estranged from God (10). This, by interpretation, suggests that many believed that many cancer diseases in the Nigerian society are afflictions from God.

Furthermore, the opinion of the surveyed religious leaders and seminarians on socioeconomic factors being responsible for having cancer is also insightful. Some of them believed that poverty and wealth can make one to develop cancer diseases. However, and fortunately, the evidenced-based medical risk factors of cancer (such as genetic factors, radiation exposure, poison, toxic drugs, etc.) were known by many of the respondents in this study; this shows that many of them acknowledged that cancers can be cause by biological, physical and chemical factors.

Conclusion

In conclusion, many of the surveyed religious leaders and seminarians were of the opinion that cancer is mainly caused by biological, physical and chemical factors; however, some of them still have the belief that socioeconomic and supernatural factors are the causes of cancers in the Nigerian society.

Acknowledgments

This study was self-funded. Authors have no conflict of interest to declare. This chapter was also a revised version of an earlier publication of the authors (11).

References

[1] Morounke SG, Ayorinde JB, Benedict AO, Adedayo FF, Adewale FO, et al. Epidemiology and incidence of common cancers in Nigeria. J Cancer Biol Res 2017;5(3):1105.

[2] Jemal A, Siegel R, Ward E, Murray T, Xu J, Smigal C, et al. Cancer statistics, 2006. Cancer J Clin 2006;56(2):106-30.

[3] Jemal A, Bray F, Center MM, Ferlay J, Ward E, Forman D. Global Cancer statistics. CA Cancer J Clin 2011;61(2):69-90.

[4] Kene TS, Odige VI, Yusufu LMD, Yusuf BO, Shehu SM, Kase JT. Pattern of presentation and survival of breast cancer in a teaching hospital in North Western Nigeria. Oman Med J 2010;25(2):104-7.

[5] Kalu M, Matthew A, Rajan B. Impact of socioeconomic factors in delaying reporting and late-stage presentation among patients with cervix cancer in a major cancer hospital in South India. Asian Pacific J Cancer Prev 9(4):589-94.

[6] Ukwenya AY, Yusufu LD, Nmadu PD, Garba ES, Ahmed A. Delayed treatment of symptomatic breast cancer: The experience from Kaduna. S Afr J Surg 2008;46(4):106-10.

[7] Adesunkanmi AR, Lawal OO, Adelusola KK, Durosimi MA. The severity, outcome and challenges of breast cancer in Nigeria. Breast 2006;15(3):399-409.

[8] Ibrahim NA, Oludara MA. Socio-demographic factors and reasons associated with delay in breast cancer presentation: A study in Nigerian women. Breast 2012;21(3):416-8.

[9] Badru AI, Kanmodi KK. Palliative care awareness amongst religious leaders and seminarians: A Nigerian study. Pan Afr Med J 2017;28:259.

[10] Merriam-Webster Dictionary. Sin. URL: https://www.merriam-webster.com/dictionary/sin.

[11] Badru AI, Kanmodi KK, Ogundipe PA, Owadokun AM, Adesina MA. Opinions of Nigerian religious leaders and seminarians on what causes cancer: A short report. J Altern Med Res 2019;11(2):165-7.

In: Nigeria: Perspectives of Health
Editors: Ariel Tenenbaum et al.
ISBN: 978-1-53618-090-9

Chapter 3

AWARENESS AND PERCEIVED NEED OF NIGERIANS ON THE RESTORATIVE TREATMENT FOR A DEFECTIVE TOOTH: A SCHOOL SURVEY

Amidu O Sulaiman[1,2], BDS, FMCDS, Kehinde K Kanmodi[1,2,*], BDS and Babatunde A Amoo[2], BSc, MPH

[1]Department of Restorative Dentistry, Faculty of Dentistry, University of Ibadan, Ibadan

[2]Cephas Health Research Initiative Inc, Ibadan, Nigeria

ABSTRACT

In this chapter we try to determine the awareness rate of students in the University of Ibadan campus on restorative dental treatment and also explore their perceived needs for a dental restoration. Methods: Data of surveyed 668 University of Ibadan students was used in this study. Study

* Corresponding Author's Email: kanmodikehinde@yahoo.com.

tool was a well-structured self-administered questionnaire. Analysis was done using the SPSS version 16 software. Results: The majority (55.2%) of the respondents were within the age range of 21-25 years, 51.3% were females, and 76.8% were Yorubas. The majority (96.9%) were aware of a dentist, while only 34.1% had ever visited a dentist in their life time. Only 14.22% had missing teeth, 17.7% had broken teeth, while 19.5% had discolored teeth. The majority (82.3%) were aware that a missing tooth can be restored. Only 47 out of the 130 respondents who had a discolored tooth felt the need to get a dental restoration. Only 115 out of 415 respondents who had a broken tooth felt the need to get a dental restoration. Removable denture is the most popularly known (36.7%) dental restorative device among the respondents. Conclusions: This study revealed a very high awareness rate of a dentist among students of the University of Ibadan. Many of these students had defective teeth that needed restoration; however many did not perceive the need to get them restored. The authors recommend the need for education and awareness on the benefits of good oral health status.

INTRODUCTION

The teeth constitute an important part of the human body that aids in mastication, phonation, and aesthetics (1). Deviation from the normal state of health of a tooth can result into a diseased state and pain (2-5). This could arise from insults to the tooth (2, 3), like trauma, bacterial action, erosive chemicals, heat, among others (4, 5), causing dental diseases like tooth wear lesions, pulpitis, pulpal necrosis, periapical abscess, pain and ultimately tooth loss (2, 6).

The literature had reported a significant prevalence of dental diseases among different Nigerian populations and across different age groups and socio-economic strata (7-10); thus making it a public health problem in Nigeria. Public awareness on oral health had also been well documented, and had been found to be increasing over the years (9-11). Despite this gradual increase in the awareness rate on oral health in Nigeria, a high prevalence of dental disease is still seen among Nigerians (10, 12). This has been attributed to a number of contributing factors including ignorance, anxiety of getting dental treatments, poverty, unperceived need for dental care, and extremely high population – dentist ratio (13-19).

Ignorance about the possibility of restorative treatment for a diseased tooth has been found to be high among lay people (13, 14), causing many of them to suffer intractable tooth ache, poor quality of life, and anodontia (14). Inability to perceive and attend to dental health needs early had also been found to be low among the lay Nigerian adult populations (15), making many of them to present late at the dental clinic when their dental diseases had already developed complications requiring higher treatment costs (15). Anxiety for dental treatment also had been well studied among different populations (16). As a matter of fact, some dentally anxious individuals often delay visiting a dental surgery for a long period of time, causing detrimental effects on their dental health conditions which in turn make their dental treatment needs more complex due to the complications that would have arisen (16). All these problems – ignorance, anxiety of dental treatment, and unperceived needs, are psychosocial factors that could be solved through oral health education (13, 20, 21).

The problems of the socio-economic deprived population – dentist ratio and high poverty rate in the country are demographic and economic problems that could be solved by the government (13, 22). Research has shown that a number of fruitful efforts, over the years, had been made by the government in this regard, to reduce the intensity of these two problems (23, 24). However, more still needs to be done in making comprehensive dental health care more accessible for the Nigerian masses (13, 22).

After thorough search of the literature, the authors observed scanty literature on the awareness of Nigerian adults on the restorative treatment options for a defective tooth, and also on their perceived need for a dental restoration (9, 25). Also, the majority of the available studies in this area were conducted amongst the health professionals and their trainees (9, 25, 26). To the best of the authors' knowledge, no published research data exist on the awareness rate and perceived needs of the University of Ibadan students on restorative dental treatment. This study aims to determine the level of awareness of the students on the University of Ibadan campus on restorative dental treatment and also to explore their perceived needs for a dental restoration.

OUR STUDY

This cross-sectional study was conducted in accordance with the Helsinki Declaration. Ethical clearance to carry out this study was officially obtained from the Ministry of Education, Ibadan, Nigeria. The study was conducted among students of the University of Ibadan. This tertiary institution is the premier university of the country and she is situated within the city of Ibadan, Nigeria. This school had a total of twelve (12) academic faculties (see Figure 1), with each faculty running both undergraduate and postgraduate academic program.

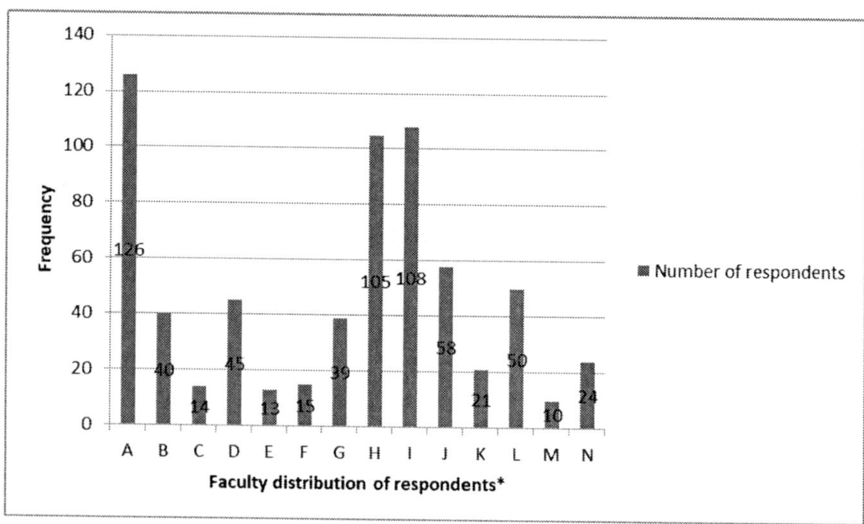

Keywords: A= Faculty of Veterinary Medicine; B= Faculty of Pharmacy; C= Faculty of Law; C= Faculty of Science; D= Faculty of Arts; E= Faculty of Public Health; F= Faculty of Agriculture; G= Faculty of Social Sciences; H= Faculty of Basic Medical Sciences; I= Faculty of Clinical Sciences; J= Faculty of Dentistry; K= Faculty of Technology; L= Faculty of Education; N= Faculty not indicated.

Figure 1. Faculty distribution of respondents.

The study tool for this present study was a well-structured four-sectioned pre-tested questionnaire, which was adapted from a similar study (9). The first section obtained information on the socio-economic attributes of the participants. The second section obtained information about participants' awareness of a dental surgeon, and the possibility of restoration of a defective or missing tooth. The third section obtained information about participants' awareness of common dental restorations. The fourth section obtained information about participants' knowledge of the use of the dental restorations mentioned earlier in the third section.

Participant's selection was based on lack of exposure to clinical training in dentistry. Based on this criterion, all bona fide students of the University of Ibadan were considered eligible, except for those dental students that have started the clinical phase of their training in dentistry and the senior medical students (i.e., those medical students in the clinical phase of their study program) who had rotated through clinical postings in dentistry.

A sample of 700 students was interviewed in this study via our study tool (i.e., a self-administered questionnaire). Study participants were approached in their classrooms and dormitories. The aims and objectives of the study were clearly explained to them, and they were also informed about the confidentiality of their participation. Verbal informed consent was sought from each participant before being issued a questionnaire to fill. Only 676 participants returned their questionnaires filled, of which 8 were discarded during data cleaning process. Data collection process was done from October to December, 2014.

Data analysis was done using the SPSS version 16 software. Frequencies of variables were illustrated using tables and a chart. Tests of association between variables were done using the Chi-square test and a p-value of <0.05 was considered to be of statistical significance.

FINDINGS

Out of the 700 persons recruited for this study, only 676 responded, giving a response rate of 96.6%. Table 1 shows the socio-demographic attributes of the participants. The majority (55.2%) were within the age range of 21-25 years, 51.3% were females, 81.6% were Christians, while 76.8% were from the Yoruba tribe. Figure 1 illustrates the faculty distribution of the respondents. About one-fifth (18.9%) of our respondents were students from the Faculty of Veterinary Medicine.

Table 1. Socio-demographic attributes of respondents

Characteristics (n=668)	N	%
*Age**		
16 – 20	205	30.7
21 – 25	369	55.2
26 – 30	64	9.6
31 – 35	6	0.9
>35	8	1.2
Not specified	16	2.4
Gender		
Male	319	47.8
Female	343	51.3
Not specified	6	0.9
Religion		
Islam	110	16.5
Christianity	545	81.6
Traditional	2	0.3
Others	5	0.7
Not specified	6	0.9
Tribe		
Yoruba	513	76.8
Igbo	84	12.6
Hausa	5	0.7
Others	58	8.7
Not specified	8	1.2

n=total number of respondents in this study; N= total number of respondents in each category; *Age was reported in years.

Table 2 shows the rate of awareness of the dentist and the possibility of restoration of a defective tooth among our respondents. The majority (96.9%) of them were aware of a dentist, however only 34.1% had never visited a dentist in their life time. Only 14.22% had a missing tooth, 17.7% had a broken tooth, while 19.5% had a discoloured tooth. The majority (82.3%) were aware that a missing tooth can be restored.

Table 2. Awareness of respondents about a dentist and the possibility of the restoration of a defective tooth

Variables	Yes (%)	No (%)	NR (%)
Do you know who a dentist is?	647 (96.9)	19 (2.8)	2 (0.3)
Have you ever visited a dentist before?	228 (34.1)	428 (64.1)	9 (0.13)
Have you had any restoration placed on your tooth before?	76 (11.4)	588 (88.0)	4 (0.6)
Do you have a missing tooth?	95 (14.2)	569 (85.2)	4 (0.6)
Are you aware of replacement of a missing tooth in the mouth?	550 (82.3)	111 (16.6)	7 (1.0)
Do you have a broken tooth?	118 (17.7)	547 (81.9)	3 (0.4)
Do you know if a broken tooth can be restored?	412 (61.7)	192 (28.7)	62 (9.3)
Do you have a discoloured tooth?	130 (19.5)	521 (78.0)	17 (2.5)
Do you know if a discoloured tooth can be restored?	328 (49.1)	286 (42.8)	54 (8.1)
Has anybody advised you to restore/replace a tooth before?	115 (17.2)	530 (79.3)	23 (3.4)

NR= No response.

Table 3. Comparison between respondents' dental problems, and perceived need for a dental restoration

		Have you ever felt the need to restore/replace a tooth at any time? **			
		Yes	No	Total	p – value (X^2)
Do you have a discoloured tooth? **	Yes	47	81	128	<0.0001
	No	67	437	504	
	Total	114	518	632	
Do you have a broken tooth? **	Yes	50	68	118	<0.0001
	No	85	460	525	
	Total	115	528	643	
Do you have a missing tooth? **	Yes	45	50	95	<0.0001
	No	68	479	547	
	Total	113	529	642	

**Not all respondents gave a response to this variable, hence missing values were not computed in this statistics.

Table 3 shows statistically significant relationships between respondents' dental problems, and perceived need for a dental restoration. Only 47 out of the 130 respondents who had a discoloured tooth felt the need to get a dental restoration (see Tables 2-3). Only 115 out of 415 respondents who had a broken tooth felt the need to get a dental restoration (see Tables 2-3.)

Table 4. Comparison between the awareness and knowledge of respondents on the specific use of the common dental restorative devices

Restorative devices	Awareness*			Knowledge of use*			p – value (X^2)
	Yes	No	NS	Yes	No	IDK	
Removable denture	283	301	63	245	42	360	<0.0001
Bridge	237	324	84	123	108	414	<0.0001
Crown	333	241	72	198	64	384	<0.0001

NS= Not sure; IDK= I don't know; *Missing values were not computed in this analysis.

Table 4 shows the comparison between the awareness and the knowledge of respondents on the specific use of the common restorative devices. Only 245 out of the 283 respondents who had heard of a removable denture knew its use. Removable denture is the most popularly known (36.7%) dental restorative device among our respondents.

DISCUSSION

Dental health can be described as the state of freedom from diseases affecting the teeth (27). Whenever there is a significant insult to a tooth, dental disease sets in. Dental diseases, such as tooth loss, tooth discolouration, and pathologic tooth fracture, can negatively affect an individual's quality of life (28, 29).

Individuals with dental diseases tend to suffer from social inequalities (29). Unfortunately, many of those with dental diseases have been found to carry these problems along with their day-to-day activities while being ignorant of the possibility of having restorations done on these defective teeth (9, 12, 14). Furthermore, some of them suffer from speech and masticatory difficulties of varying degree of severity, depending on the stage of the dental disease progression (30-32).

A way to nib the progression of dental diseases and its complications is to seek for a professional dental care (15). The aspect of dentistry that deals with the restoration of diseased tooth is called restorative dentistry. The various possible restorative treatment options for a diseased tooth include dental filling, crown, veneer, denture, bridge, dental implant, among others.

Quite a number of studies had been published on the awareness rate of oral health and the prevalence of perceived oral health needs among different Nigerian populations (9-11, 13-15). However, to the best of the authors' knowledge, no published article had reported data on these subject areas amongst the population of the University of Ibadan students. The need for relevant research data on the prevalence of perceived restorative dental needs and the level of awareness of University of Ibadan students on restorative dental treatment options informed the authors to conduct this present study.

In this present study, the authors observed that the majority (96.9%) of the respondents were aware of the dentist (see Table 2). Unfortunately, many (64.1%) of them had never visited a dentist in their life time. This finding is slightly similar to that reported by Sulaiman and Kanmodi (9) in a study where they reported an awareness rate of 99.0% among some surveyed nursing students in Ibadan. In their study, they observed that the majority (78.5%) of their respondents had never visited a dentist in their life time; however this rate was higher than the one observed (64.1%) in this study. Overall, this shows that many tertiary students in Ibadan do not visit a dentist for regular dental check-ups, despite the high awareness rate of the dentist among them. Many of the respondents in this study had missing, fractured, and discoloured teeth; however not all of them have had them restored/replaced. This may be due to many factors, some of which may include ignorance, stress of visiting a dentist, anxiety, and financial limitations (13, 14, 17, 19, 33).

Some of the respondents who had fractured teeth did not see any need to get those teeth restored. This may be due to ignorance of the possible complications associated with tooth fracture. The complications that could arise from a fractured tooth include pulpal necrosis, periapical abscess, periapical cyst, dentoalveolar abscess, tissue space infections, cavernous sinus thrombophlebitis, amongst others. This finding reveals a necessitating need to appropriately educate this population group on the socioeconomic and health benefits of seeking early treatment of a fractured tooth.

This study also showed that removable denture is the most popularly known restorative device among the respondents in this study. This finding is similar to that reported among a population of surveyed nursing students in Ibadan (9). Authors suggest that the relatively low cost of removable dentures, amongst other restorations, may be the most likely reason why removable denture is the most popular dental restoration among this study population.

Quite a lot of the respondents in this study did not know about the use of the common types of dental restorative devices. This suggests that many of them had limited knowledge of the different restorative options they could seek for regarding their defective teeth. This calls for the need to educate them on this area.

This study has its limitations. It did not explore the reasons why some study participants had not visited a dentist in their life time. It also did not enquire into the purpose of the past dental visits of the respondents. This study surveyed a single institution; hence data of students in other tertiary institutions were not captured.

CONCLUSION

To the best of the authors' knowledge, this study is the first study that ever determined and explored awareness rate and perceived needs for restorative dental treatment amongst the University of Ibadan students, respectively. Most of the available published studies that had been conducted in this area only surveyed Nigerian health professionals and trainees (9, 25, 26). In this study, we observed a very high awareness rate of a dentist amongst students of the University of Ibadan. Furthermore, many of them had never visited a dentist in their life time; hence they lacked adequate knowledge about their oral health status. Some of them had fractured, discoloured, and/or missing teeth that need restoration, but had not got them restored. This shows the need to educate and encourage them to get those teeth restored before complications develop from them. Educating them about this issue is very important because many of the individuals in our environment do present late to the dentist when complications had already occurred (15).

ACKNOWLEDGMENTS

This study was conceptualized by AOS and KKK. Data collection was done by AOS and KKK. Data analysis was done by BAA and KKK. Manuscript write-up was done by AOS and KKK. All authors read and approved the manuscript. Authors have no competing interest to declare. Authors give thanks to Ms Beauty Iyioku for her technical assistance in the study. This study was self-funded.

REFERENCES

[1] Ibiyemi O, Taiwo JO. Psychosocial aspect of anterior tooth discolouration among adolescents in Igbo-ora, Southwestern Nigeria. Ann Ib Postgrad Med 2011;9(2):95-100.

[2] Hattab FN, Qudeimat MA, al-Rimawi HS. Dental discolouration: An overview. J Esthet Dent 1999;11(6):291-310.

[3] Andreasen FM, Kahler B. Pulpal response after acute dental injury in the permanent dentition: clinical implications: A review. J Endod 2015;41(3):299-308.

[4] Hanif A, Rashid H, Nasim M. Tooth surface loss revisited: classification, etiology, and management. J Res Dent 2015;3(2):37-43.

[5] Caufield PW, Griffen AL. Dental caries. An infectious and transmissible disease. Pediatr Clin North Am 2000;47(5):1001-19.

[6] Kassebaum NJ, Bernabe E, Dahiya M, Bhandari B, Murray CJL, Marcenes W. Global burden of severe tooth loss: A systematic review and meta-analysis. J Dent Res 2014; 93(7 Suppl):20S-8.

[7] Folayan MO, Adeniyi AA, Chukwumah NM, Onyejaka N, Esan AO, Sofola O, et al. Programme guidelines for promoting good oral health for children in Nigeria: a position paper. BMC Oral Health 2014;14:128. doi:10.1186/1472-6831-14-128.

[8] Oginno FO. Tooth loss in a sub-urban Nigerian population: causes and pattern of mortality revisited. Int Dent J 2005;55(1):17-23.

[9] Sulaiman AO, Kanmodi KK. Awareness of restorative dental treatment as shown by nursing students in Ibadan. J Stoma 2016;69(6):667-73.

[10] Akpata ES. Oral health in Nigeria. Int Dent J 2004;54:361-6.

[11] Peterson PE. Improvement of oral health in Africa in the 21st century: The role of WHO Global Health Programme. Dev Dent 2004;5(1):9-20.

[12] Azodo CC, Amenaghawon OP. Oral hygiene status and practices among rural dwellers. Eur J Gen Dent 2013;2(1):42-5.

[13] Olusile AO. Improving low awareness and inadequate access to oral health care in Nigeria: the role of dentists, the government & non-governmental agencies. Nig Med J 2010;51(3):134-6.

[14] Bashiru BO, Omotunde SM. Burden of oral diseases and dental treatment needs of an urban population in Port Harcourt, Rivers State, Nigeria. Eur J Gen Dent 2014;3(2):125-8.

[15] Ajayi DM, Abiodun-Solanke IM, Sulaiman AO, Ekhalufoh EF. A retrospective study of traumatic injuries to teeth at a Nigerian tertiary hospital. Nig J Clin Pract 2012; 15(3):320-5.

[16] Armfield JM, Heaton LJ. Management of fear and anxiety in the dental clinic: A review. Aust Dent J 2013;58(4):390-407.

[17] Akaji EA, Oredugba FA, Jeboda SO. Utilization of dental services among secondary school students in Lagos. Nig Dent J 2007;15(2):87-91.

[18] Udoye CI, Oginni AO, Oginni FO. Dental anxiety among patients undergoing various dental treatments in a Nigerian teaching hospital. J Contemp Dent Pract 2005;6:91-8.

[19] Timis T, Danila I. Socio-economic status and oral health. J Prev Med 2005;13:116-21.

[20] Amin M, Nyachhyon P, Elyasi M, Al-Nuaimi M. Impact of an oral health education workshop on parents' oral health knowledge, attitude, and perceived behavioural control among African immigrants. J Oral Dis 2014;2014:986745. doi:10.1155/2014/986745.

[21] Jeboda SO. Perceptive needs and oral health education. Nig Qt J Hosp Med 1998;3:187-9.

[22] Adeniyi AA, Sofola OO, Kalliecharan RV. An appraisal of the oral health care system in Nigeria. Int Dent J 2012;62:292-300.

[23] Federal Ministry of Health. National health policy and strategy to achieve oral health for all Nigerians (draft). Abuja: FMoH, 1999.

[24] Federal Ministry of Health. National oral health policy (draft). Abuja: FMoH, 2010.

[25] Azodo CC, Ehizele AO, Umoh A, Ojehanon PI, Akhionbare O, Okechukwu R, et al. Perceived oral health status and treatment needs of dental auxillaries. Libyan J Med 2010; 5(1):4859. doi:10.3402/ljm.v5i0.4859.

[26] Oyetola EO, Oyewole T, Adedigba M, Aregbesola ST, Umezudike K, Adewale A. Knowledge and awareness of medical doctors, medical students and nurses about dentistry in Nigeria. Pan Afr Med J 2016;23:172. doi:10.11604/pamj. 2016.23.172.7696.

[27] World Health Organization. Fact sheet 318, 2010. Data query. URL: http://www.who.int/mediacentre/factsheets/fs318/en/index.html.

[28] Ayo-Yusuf OA, Motioba DP, Rantao M. The dental profession: promoting psychosocial well-being and not just treatment of oral disease. S Afr Dent J 2015;70(2):46-7.

[29] Willis MS, Esquela CW, Schacht RN. Social perceptions of individuals missing upper front teeth. Percept Mot Skills 2008;106(2):423-35..

[30] Stelzle F, Ugrinovic B, Knipfer C, Bocklet T, Noth E, Schuster M, et al. Automatic, computer-based speech assessment on edentulous patients with and without complete dentures – preliminary results. J Oral Rehabil 2010;37(3):209-16.

[31] Ichikawa J, Komoda J, Horiuchi M, Matsumoto N. Influence of alterations in the oral environment on speech production. J Oral Rehabil 1995;22(4):295-9.

[32] Zlataric DK, Celebic A. Factors related to patients' general satisfaction with removable partial dentures: a stepwise multiple regression analysis. Int J Prosthodont 2008; 21(1):86-8.

[33] Locker D, Ford J. Evaluation of an area-based measure as an indicator of inequalities in oral health. Commun Dent Oral Epidemiol 1994;22:80-5.

In: Nigeria: Perspectives of Health
Editors: Ariel Tenenbaum et al.
ISBN: 978-1-53618-090-9

Chapter 4

THE ROLE OF FEAR OF MENTAL ILLNESS ON ACADEMIC PERFORMANCE OF NIGERIAN MEDICAL STUDENTS

Kehinde K Kanmodi[1,*], BDS
and Bello Almu[2], BSc, MPPA
[1]Cephas Health Research Initiative Inc, Sokoto
[2]Department of Sociology, Usmanu Danfodiyo University, Sokoto, Nigeria

ABSTRACT

There is a popular belief in the Nigerian society that reading too much can result in mental illness. Interestingly, virtually no research literature had recorded any relationship between this belief and academic performance of Nigerian students. *Objectives:* To evaluate the impact of the belief that reading too much can cause mental illness on the academic performance of Nigerian students. Study group: The final year medical students of the Usmanu Danfodiyo University, Sokoto, Nigeria. Methods: A cross-section of 60 final year medical students was interviewed using a

* Corresponding Author's Email: kanmodikehinde@yahoo.com.

self-administered anonymous questionnaire. The questionnaire obtained information from the participants on their socio-demographic characteristics, academic records, and beliefs on reading too much to be a cause of mental illness. Data obtained were analyzed using the SPSS version 16 software. *Results*: The mean (±SD) age of the respondents was 26.05 (±4.34) years, and the majority (83.3%) of them were males. Less than one-tenth (6.7%) of them reported that they had excellent performance in their current study programme. A higher proportion of the females, when compared to the males, were of the mind-set that too much reading is dangerous to the brain (6/10 [60%] versus 16/50 [32%], p-value = 0.533). Also, a higher proportion of those that did not believe that reading too much could cause mental illness had a very good to excellent academic record in their current academic program, when compared to those with such belief (12/39 [30.8%] versus 3/13 [23.1%], p-value = 0.409). *Conclusion*: Students who did not believe that they can develop mental illness as a result of reading too much generally had better academic performance than those that had such belief.

INTRODUCTION

Education is a powerful tool for the attainment and sustenance of development of any nation. For any nation to develop, her citizens need to be properly educated and well informed. More importantly, it is not sufficient for the citizens of a nation to just attend school, but getting the best from school education should be the main focus. In Nigeria, a lot of individuals are in school, however only a small fraction of them are getting the best from school education (1). There are many factors that limit Nigerian students from getting the best from school education. Some of these factors include poverty, terrorism, and socio-cultural beliefs, among others (2-5).

If we focus on socio-cultural beliefs, we will find many factors limiting the proper utilization of educational opportunities among Nigerian students. For example, it is a popular belief in some Nigerian societies that educating a girl-child is a sheer waste of time, because a girl child is presumed to end up as a housewife when married (3). This belief had hindered many girls from getting the best from school education (3). From our observation, there is also a popular societal belief that reading too much can cause mental illness; this belief had made many people to embrace academic mediocrity on account of fears of developing mental illnesses that may arise from rigorous pursuit of academic prowess. After extensive literature search, we found that virtually no literature had recorded any relationship between this belief and academic performance of Nigerian students.

It will be of many benefits to the Nigerian society if the impact of the fear of developing mental illness from reading too much can be measured among Nigerian students. This study aims to evaluate the impact of this belief on the academic performance of Nigerian students, using the final year medical students in Sokoto State, Nigeria, as a case study. Conducting this kind of study among this peculiar population group (i.e., medical students) is of high significance, being that this population group is expected to be more medically knowledgeable about the medical causes of mental illness than the lay populations. Hence, the findings made from this study will give a projection of what may obtain of such among the lay populations.

OUR STUDY

This study was a cross-sectional study conducted under the guidelines of the Helsinki declaration on research involving human subjects. The study population was the medical students studying at the medical school of the Usmanu Danfodiyo University (UDU), Sokoto Metropolis, Sokoto State, Nigeria. This university (i.e., UDU) is the home to the one and only medical school in the entire Sokoto State. This school runs a six-year medical degree program. This program has two phases, which are the pre-clinical and the clinical phases; those students in the 1st, 2nd, and 3rd undergraduate years (UGYs) are in the pre-clinical phase while those in the 4th, 5th, and 6th UGYs are in the clinical phase. Those medical students that are in the clinical phase of their medical program are domiciled within the Usmanu Danfodiyo University Teaching Hospital (UDUTH), while those in the preclinical phase are domiciled within the university campuses. This hospital is a tertiary hospital affiliated to the UDU. Both the hospital and the university campuses are situated within Sokoto metropolis. The study instrument was a well-structured questionnaire designed by the authors. The questionnaire had three sections:

- The 1st section obtained information on the socio-demographic characteristics of the participants;
- The 2nd section obtained information on the participants' beliefs regarding reading too much to be a cause of mental illness;
- And the 3rd section obtained information on the participants' academic records

Authors developed some two criteria for the participants' selection. Below are those criteria:

- Willingness to participate in the study
- Completion of clinical postings in Psychiatry

The justification for including the completion of postings in Psychiatry as part of the eligibility criteria was that Psychiatry is a medical specialty that deals with the management of mental illnesses; hence, this will ensure that all subjects are averagely knowledgeable about the causes and risk factors of mental illnesses before participating.

Based on these eligibility criteria highlighted above, only those medical students in their 6th UGY (n = 98) could participate in this study.

The eligible medical students (i.e., those in their 6th UGY) were approached at their lecture hall and dormitories. They were informed about the purpose of the study, and that their participation is strictly voluntary and confidential. Only those that gave verbal informed consent to participate in the study were given an anonymous questionnaire to fill and return. Participants' selection was done using simple random sampling technique. Out of the 65 questionnaires administered, only 60 were returned filled.

All the retuned questionnaires (n = 60) were used for this study; none was discarded because they were all appropriately filled. Data was analyzed using the SPSS version 16 software. Frequency distributions of all variables were determined and Chi-square test was used to compare relationships between the qualitative variables with a p-value of <0.005 considered to be of statistical significance. The results obtained from the analysis were presented using tables and charts.

Table 1. Socio-demographic characteristics of respondents

Characteristics	N (%)
Gender	
Male	50 (83.3)
Female	10 (16.7)
Mean (±SD) age*	26.05 (±4.34)
Tribe	
Yoruba	11 (18.3)
Hausa	39 (65.0)
Igbo	1 (1.7)
Others	8 (13.3)
Not mentioned	1 (1.7)
Marital status	
Single	52 (86.7)
Married	8 (13.3)
Religion	
Christianity	9 (15.0)
Islam	61 (85.0)

*Age was recorded in years; N = Total number of respondents in each category.

FINDINGS

The mean (±SD) age of the respondents was 26.05 (±4.34) years. The majority of them were single (86.7%), and in the male gender (83.3%) category (see Table 1).

Table 2. Comparison between the depths of belief of the respondents on "reading too much" to be dangerous to the brain with the frequency of sitting attempts for their O' level examination

Variable		Too much reading is dangerous for the brain (n = 60)						X2
		SD	D	U	A	SA	Total	p-value, df
How many times did you sit for your O' level examination before you passed all the 5 compulsory subjects you needed to secure admission for your current study programme?	Once	6 (10.0)	14 (23.3)	3 (5.0)	14 (23.3)	3 (5.0)	40 (66.7)	0.730, df = 20
	Twice	3 (5.0)	4 (6.7)	3 (5.0)	2 (3.3)	1 (1.7)	13 (21.7)	
	Thrice	1 (1.7)	0 (0.0)	1 (1.7)	1 (1.7)	1 (1.7)	4 (6.7)	
	Four times	0 (0.0)	1 (1.7)	0 (0.0)	0 (0.0)	0 (0.0)	1 (1.7)	
	Five times	0 (0.0)	1 (1.7)	0 (0.0)	0 (0.0)	0 (0.0)	1 (1.7)	
	>5 times	1 (1.7)	0 (0.0)	0 (0.0)	0 (0.0)	0 (0.0)	1 (1.7)	
	Total	11 (18.3)	20 (33.3)	7 (11.7)	17 (28.3)	5 (8.3)	60 (100.0)	

SD = Strongly disagree; D = Disagree; U = Undecided; A = Agree; SA = Strongly agree.

Table 3. Comparison between the beliefs of the respondents on "reading too much" to be a mental illness risk factor with their academic performance

Variable		Reading too much can make me run mad (n = 60)*						X2
		SD	D	U	A	SA	Total	p-value, df
So far in your current academic program, what is the rating of your academic performance?	Average	5 (83.3)	6 (10.0)	2 (3.3)	2 (3.3)	2 (3.3)	17 (28.3)	0.409, df = 12
	Good	7 (11.7)	9 (15.0)	4 (6.7)	6 (10.0)	0 (0.0)	26 (43.3)	
	Very good	6 (10.0)	3 (5.0)	0 (0.0)	2 (3.3)	0 (0.0)	11 (18.3)	
	Excellent	2 (3.3)	1 (1.7)	0 (0.0)	0 (0.0)	1 (1.7)	4 (6.7)	
	Total	20 (33.3)	19 (31.7)	6 (10.0)	10 (16.7)	3 (5.0)	58 (96.7)	

*Data of two respondents were not computed because they gave no complete response to the variables cross-tabulated.

SD = Strongly disagree; D = Disagree; U = Undecided; A = Agree; SA = Strongly agree.

The majority (66.7%) of the respondents made a minimum of credit pass in all the 5 compulsory subjects needed to secure their admission into their current medical programme in a sitting (see Table 2). Also, less than one-tenth (6.7%) of the respondents reported that they had excellent performance in their current study programme (see Table 3).

A higher proportion of the females, when compared to the males, were of the mind-set that too much of reading is dangerous to the brain (6/10 [60%] versus 16/50 [32%], p-value = 0.533) (see figure 1). Furthermore, a higher proportion of those respondents that did not belief that reading too much is dangerous to the brain passed their O' level entrance examination to the university at one sitting when compared to those that believed the opposite (20/21 [95.2%] versus 17/23 [73.9%]) (see Table 2).

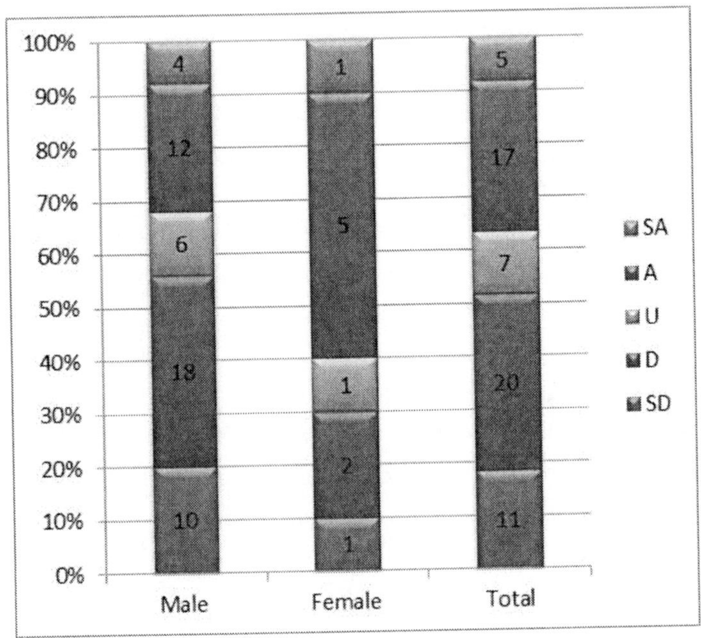

p-value = 0.533, df = 4 (X^2).

SD = Strongly disagree; D = Disagree; U = Undecided; A = Agree; SA = Strongly agree.

Figure 1. Response of the respondents to the statement: Too much reading is dangerous to the brain.

Lastly, a higher proportion of those that did not believe that reading too much could cause mental illness had a very good to excellent academic record in their current academic program, when compared to those with such belief (12/39 [30.8%] versus 3/13 [23.1%], p-value = 0.409) (see Table 3).

DISCUSSION

Madness can be defined as a state of severe mental illness (6). Mental illness can be described as a health condition involving changes in thinking, emotion or behaviour (or a combination of these) (7). The risk factors for mental illness among school-age individuals are diverse (8). However, some school-related risk factors that could cause mental illnesses among these individuals include adverse learning environment, difficulties at school, and lack of educational opportunities (8).

It is noteworthy that the impact of Nigerian socio-cultural beliefs on mental illness on formal education had been under-explored. For instance, and to the best of the authors' knowledge, no available study had reported the impacts of such beliefs on the academic performance of tertiary school students. The rationale for conducting this study was to explore the impact of the fear of developing mental illness as a result of reading too much.

In this study, it is alarming that despite the level of medical knowledge of the respondents on the aetiology and risk factors of mental illness, yet a significant proportion of them still believed that reading too much could cause mental illness. If this kind of belief was found to be as this common among final year medical students, how much more the medical students in lower classes as well as those students in the non-medical disciplines. Furthermore, this belief was found to tell negatively on the academic performance of those medical students that believed in such. By implication, it could be said that quite many of them had not benefitted maximally from medical education due to this belief.

In the nearest future, the respondents in this present study will hopefully graduate as a medical doctor, and start working as clinicians.

Clinical practice requires continual medical education. A clinician who desires to be of relevance in the society needs to keep updating his/her medical knowledge from time to time. To be up to date in the current trends of patient management, a clinician has to passionately embrace lifetime studying. From this juncture, it is good to recall that many of the surveyed medical students believed that reading too much could make them develop mental illness. This may suggest that some of them may possibly not want to further their medical education after concluding their medical programme, due to the heavier academic workload in postgraduate studies, which will demand more intensive studying of books.

For a nation to be strong, the factors limiting the maximal utilization of her citizens on educational pursuits need to be successfully eradicated. In this study, we found out that the fear of developing mental illness from reading too much is a factor limiting the surveyed medical students from having better academic performance in their current study program. Based on this finding, it could be said further that students in other academic disciplines will most likely be experiencing similar problems, telling negatively on their academic performance likewise.

However, this study has its limitation. This study did not survey the medical students in lower classes as well as those in other Nigerian medical schools; this informs the need to conduct a bigger study on this subject matter. Also, this study did not enquire into the reasons why the respondents believed that reading too much could cause mental illness; hence, conducting a qualitative study to explore the reasons behind this belief among medical students will be of benefit. From the findings made in this research, authors would like to recommend the following:

- Proper education and counselling of medical students, as well as the entire public, on the evidence-based causes of mental illness
- A need for research to explore the degree of impact of the belief that reading too much could cause mental illness on the academic performance of Nigerian students from the secondary to the tertiary level of education

- Disabusing the minds of Nigerian youths from the beliefs that reading too much could make them develop mental illness

In conclusion, the wrong belief that reading too much is dangerous to the brain had contributed negatively to the academic performance of the surveyed Nigerian doctors-to-be. Academic diligence is not a risk factor for mental illness; rather it boosts one's memory status, and help to reduce one's risk of developing neurodegenerative diseases like Alzheimer's diseases (9). Proper public education needs to be done on the proven risk factors of mental illness. It will also be very helpful to the Nigerian society if a survey could be conducted to assess the extent of the damage made by this popularly observed belief among Nigerian youths.

Acknowledgments

This study was funded by the authors. Authors appreciate the kind assistance of Mr Tajudeen Musbau, a medical student of the UDU, during the data collection process. Also, this chapter was a revised version of an earlier publication of the authors (10).

References

[1] UNESCO. Education and literacy. URL: http://uis.unesco.org/en/country/NG.

[2] Amzat IH. The effect of poverty on education in Nigeria: Obstacles and solutions. Oida Int J Sustain Dev 2010;1(4):55-72.

[3] Eweniyi GB, Usman IG. Perception of parents on the socio-cultural, religious and economic factors affecting girl-child education in the northern parts of Nigeria. Afr Res Rev 2013;7(3):58-74.

[4] Abdulrasheed O, Onuselogu A, Obioma UG. Effects of insurgency on universal basic education in Borno State of Nigeria. Am J Educ Res 2015;3(4):490-494.

[5] Bamigboye G, Ede A, Adeyemi G. Impact of economic crisis on education: a case study of Southwest Nigeria. Proceedings of INTED2016 Conference 7th-9th March 2016, Valencia, Spain, 2893-6. ISBN: 978-84-608-5617-7.

[6] Merriam-Webster. Madness. URL: https://www.merriam-webster.com/dictionary/madness.

[7] American Psychiatric Association. What is mental illness? URL: https://www.psychiatry.org/patients-families/what-is-mental-illness.

[8] World Health Organization. Risks to mental health: an overview of vulnerabilities and risk factors. Background paper by WHO Secretariat for the Development of a Comprehensive Mental Health Action Plan, 2012.

[9] Healthline. Alzheimer's disease prevention. URL: https://www.healthline.com/health/alzheimers-disease-prevention.

[10] Kanmodi KK, Almu B. Impact of fear of mental illness on academic performance: A case study of Sokoto medical students, Nigeria. Int J Child Health Hum Dev 2019;12(2):99-104.

In: Nigeria: Perspectives of Health
Editors: Ariel Tenenbaum et al.
ISBN: 978-1-53618-090-9

Chapter 5

DO EXPECTANT MOTHERS IN SOKOTO CITY ACTUALLY WANT THE HBV VACCINE?

Catherine Fidelis[1,2], BPharm,
Kehinde K Kanmodi[2,*], BDS
and Johnson Olajolumo[3], MBBS

[1]Department of Pharmacy, Usmanu Danfodiyo University Teaching Hospital, Sokoto, Nigeria
[2]Cephas Health Research Initiative Inc, Sokoto, Nigeria
[3]Department of Internal Medicine, Obafemi Awolowo University Teaching Hospital, Ile-Ife, Nigeria

ABSTRACT

Hepatitis B viral infection is a killer disease that can be prevented through proper vaccination. This study aims to determine the awareness and acceptance rates of hepatitis B vaccination by pregnant women in Sokoto City, Nigeria. Methods: A cross-section of 330 pregnant women was surveyed in this study using an interviewer-administered questionnaire. The questionnaire obtained information on the demographic profile,

* Correspondenceing author's Email: kanmodikehinde@yahoo.com.

hepatitis B vaccine awareness, vaccination status, and attitudes of the subjects towards hepatitis B vaccination. Data collected was analyzed using the SPSS version 20 software. Results: All the respondents were married, 40.3% of them were within the age range of 20 to 25 years, 74.8% had no source of income, and 38.5% had no formal education. Only 3.9% of the respondents were aware of hepatitis B vaccine, of which none of them had ever received the vaccine. However, more than 90% of the respondents would like to get the vaccine. Conclusions: The findings made from this study revealed a very low awareness rate on hepatitis B vaccine amongst pregnant women in Sokoto City, Nigeria. However, many of them would like to get vaccinated against HB infection.

INTRODUCTION

Hepatitis B (HB) viral infection is a potentially life-threatening liver infection that is chronically affecting about 370 million individuals globally; unfortunately, about 2 million people die of complications arising from the disease yearly (1). Hepatitis B viral infection is known to be caused by the hepatitis B virus (HBV). This virus is a double stranded DNA virus which belongs to the hepadnaviridae family. The mature HBV is spherical in shape and it has 4 different genes; these genes include the HBsAg, HBcAg, HBeAg, and the nucleocapsid which encloses the viral DNA (2-4).

In Nigeria, pregnant women constitute one of the population groups that are highly predisposed to hepatitis B infection (5). Furthermore, statistics had shown that about 14.1% of pregnant women in Nigeria are living with hepatitis B infection (5). One of the major problems associated with hepatitis B infection among pregnant women is mother-to-child transmission (MTCT) of the virus (6). Sadly, about 1 out of 10 Nigerian children are infected with hepatitis B, of which the majority of them acquired the infection through MTCT of the virus (5-7). In order to eradicate MTCT of HBV in Nigeria, the Nigerian government began HB vaccination programs in the year 2004 (2, 8); fortunately these programs are still active till date. Furthermore, impressive success rates had been recorded through these vaccination programs (9-12). However, there are still some stumbling blocks hindering the holistic success of these vaccination programs. Some of these stumbling blocks include: low awareness rate on the disease; lack of reliable cold chain in storing the vaccine; illiteracy; limited health personnel; poverty; and ignorance (7, 13).

From our literature search, we observed that different studies have determined the awareness and acceptance rates of HB vaccination among people in different geographical areas in Nigeria (14-23). Interestingly, the majority of those studies were found to have been conducted among health workers. However, we observed that only very scanty literatures were available on the awareness and acceptance rates of HB vaccination among pregnant women in Nigeria.

This study aims to: determine the awareness rate on HB vaccination; determine the acceptance rate of HB vaccination; and also explore the factors that might have influenced the choice of pregnant women in Sokoto City, northwestern Nigeria, on accepting hepatitis B vaccine. This study is of high significance, as the study will provide the first literature exploring the factors influencing the choice of acceptance of HB vaccine among pregnant women in Sokoto City, northwestern Nigeria.

OUR STUDY

This study was a cross-sectional survey of pregnant women attending the antenatal clinics of two public hospitals situated within Sokoto City, Nigeria. The names of the two surveyed hospitals were: Maryam Abacha Women and Children Hospital; and Specialist Hospital. These hospitals are owned by the Sokoto State Government, Sokoto State, Nigeria.

This study was done in accordance with the Helsinki Declaration on health research involving human subjects. Approval to conduct the study was officially obtained from the State Health Research Ethics Committee, Ministry of Health, Sokoto State, Nigeria (Ref. No: SKHREC/081/017). Permission to collect research data was also sought from the management of the participating hospitals. The identity of the study subjects were kept with strict confidentiality, during and after the study. The subjects were also given the right to decline participating in the study at any stage should they find it uncomfortable to continue. Only those that gave informed consents were recruited for the study.

The study tool was a 14-item paper questionnaire developed through literature review (24-26). The questionnaire obtained information on the demographic profile, hepatitis B vaccine awareness, vaccination status, and attitudes of each subjects toward hepatitis B vaccination. Before the above information was obtained from the subjects, the subjects were first informed about the meaning of hepatitis B in lay man terms. Also, the questionnaire was first drafted in English before being translated into Hausa: the most widely spoken local language in the study area. The translation was done by an experienced translator who is a native speaker of Hausa. The questionnaire was then back-translated into English by another translator and comparison was made for similarity, of which was found satisfactory. The questionnaire was then pretested and all necessary adjustments were made in the questionnaire to suit the purpose of the study.

The minimum sample size for this study (n=280) was determined using the Leslie formula for study population <10,000 at a HBV awareness rate of 24% derived from a previous study conducted among pregnant women in Punjab, Pakistan (24).

Within the month of December, 2017, a total of 340 pregnant women attending the antenatal clinics of the above-mentioned hospitals were approached and invited to participate in the study; only 330 women gave their consent to participate. All subjects' data were collected with the questionnaire, via face-to-face interviews. Data was analyzed using the SPSS version 20 software. The frequency distribution of all variables were determine, and comparisons between variables were done using the Chi-square test with a p-value of <0.05 set to be the level of statistical significance. Results obtained were presented using tables.

FINDINGS

Response rate was 97.1% (330/340). Four-tenth (40.3%) of the respondents were within the age range of 20 to 25 years, 44.2% had been pregnant for 1 to 3 times (aside their current pregnancy as of the time of the interview), and all (100.0%) were married. Furthermore, about two-fifth (38.5%) of the respondents had no formal education, 74.8% had no source of income, and 68.5% were married in a monogamous setting (see Table 1).

Table 1. Characteristics of the respondents

Characteristic	**Frequency (%)**
Age (in years)	
<20	56 (17.0)
20 – 25	133 (40.3)
26 – 30	91 (27.6))
31 – 35	26 (7.9)
35 – 40	19 (5.8)
>40	4 (1.2)
I do not know my age	1 (0.3)
Total number of pregnancies	
None	64 (19.4)
1 – 3	146 (44.2)
4 – 7	97 (29.4)
>7	23 (7.0)
Marital status	
Married	330 (100.0)
Educational level	
No formal education	127 (38.5)
Primary	56 (17.0)
Secondary	120 (36.4)
Tertiary	27 (8.2)
Total	330 (100.0)
Average monthly income (in Naira)	
No income	247 (74.8)
1000 – 10,000	73 (22.1)
>10,000	10 (3.0)
Family setting	
Monogamy	226 (68.5)
Polygamy	104 (31.5)

Only 3.9% of the respondents were aware of the hepatitis B vaccine. From comparisons between educational levels and awareness of respondents on the vaccine, we found that the majority (61.5%) of those that were aware of the vaccine had tertiary school education (p-value<0.0001) (see Table 2). None of the respondents had ever been vaccinated against HBV (see Table 3).

Table 2. Comparison between awareness on hepatitis B vaccine and educational level of respondents

Question	Response	Educational level of respondents					p-value (X^2)
		No formal education (N=127)	Primary (N=56)	Secondary (N=120)	Tertiary (N=27)	Total (N=330)	
Before now, have you ever heard about hepatitis B vaccine?	Yes	3 (2.4)	0 (0.0)	2 (1.7)	8 (29.6)	13 (3.9)	<0.0001, df=3
	No	124(97.6)	56(100.0)	118(98.3)	19 (70.4)	317(96.1)	
Total		127(100.0)	56(100.0)	120(100.0)	27(100.0)	330(100.0)	

N=Total number of respondents in each category; X^2=Chi square; df=Degree of freedom.

Table 3. Comparison between hepatitis B vaccination history and educational level of respondents

Question	Response	Educational level of respondents					p-value (X^2)
		No formal education (N=127)	Primary (N=56)	Secondary (N=120)	Tertiary (N=27)	Total (N=330)	X^2
Have you ever been vaccinated against HBV?	Yes	0(0.0)	0(0.0)	0(0.0)	0(0.0)	0(0.0)	***
	No	127(100.0)	56(100.0)	120(100.0)	27(100.0)	330(100.0)	
Total		127(100.0)	56(100.0)	120(100.0)	27(100.0)	330(100.0)	

N=Total number of respondents in each category; X^2=Chi square; df=Degree of freedom; ***No statistics were computed because "HAVE YOU EVER BEEN VACCINATED AGAINST HEPATITIS B BEFORE" was a constant.

Table 4 provides information on the attitudes of the respondents towards HB vaccination. The majority (94.8%) of the respondents had never been vaccinated against HB infection due to unawareness. However, more than 90% of them reported that: they would like to get the vaccine; and their husband would allow them to get vaccinated against the disease. Interestingly, the cost of HB vaccine was found to be a factor limiting the majority (63.0%) of the respondents in enrolling for HB vaccination.

Table 4. Attitudes of respondents toward hepatitis B vaccination

Question	Response	Frequency (%)
Why have you not been vaccinated against HBV?	Unaware that hepatitis B vaccine exist	313 (94.8)
	Unaware that the vaccine was important	14 (4.2)
	Do not believe that the vaccine is effective	1 (0.3)
	Do not believe that the vaccine is safe	1 (0.3)
	Religion does not permit vaccination	1 (0.3)
Would your husband allow you to be vaccinated against hepatitis B infection?	Yes	308 (93.3)
	No	18 (5.5)
	Not sure	4 (1.2)
Would the cost of the vaccine be a determinant to you been vaccinated?	Yes	208 (63.0)
	No	122 (37.0)
Do you like to be vaccinated against hepatitis B infection?	Yes	322 (97.6)
	No	5 (1.5)
	Not sure	3 (0.9)
Assuming you have hepatitis B infection, would you still allow your baby to receive anti-HBV antibodies?	Yes	325 (98.5)
	No	4 (1.2)
	Not sure	1 (0.3)
Assuming you are diagnosed to have HBV infection, would you be willing to take the drugs, which are safe, given to you by your doctor in order to prevent HBV transmission to your baby?	Yes	325 (98.5)
	No	3 (0.9)
	Not sure	2 (0.6)

HBV=Hepatitis B virus.

DISCUSSION

With the findings made in this study, it is glaring that the Nigerian government still has a long way to go for her to achieve her set goals of eradicating MTCT of HBV in Nigeria. In this study, a very low (3.9%) awareness rate on hepatitis B vaccine was recorded among the pregnant women that took part in the questionnaire; this rate is much more lower than that reported among pregnant women in other international cities (24, 26). Also, none of the respondents in this present study had ever received HB vaccination. This reveals that all of the respondents are at risk of getting infected with HB if exposed to the virus. For those among them who might have been already infected with the virus, their babies stand at high risk of contracting the viral infection through MTCT.

Interestingly, only very few respondents were aware of the HB vaccine, and none of these few had got themselves vaccinated against HBV. The reasons for non-vaccination were: vaccination against the virus was not important; the safety profile of the vaccine could not be guaranteed; and the efficacy of the vaccine could not be guaranteed. Hence, it could be assumed that some of them had been misinformed about the importance of HB vaccination.

Aside the above-mentioned factors (such as unawareness, fear of safety of HB vaccine, and doubt of efficacy of HB vaccine) hindering the respondents from getting vaccinated against HBV, objection of spouses towards enrollment for HB vaccination, religious beliefs, lack of personal income, as well as the cost of the vaccine were also considerable limiting factors.

Based on our findings, many of the respondents in this study were at high risk of contracting hepatitis B infection. This observation was made based on the socio-demographic attributes of the respondents, as many of them fell into the categories of those that were: illiterate; married in a polygamous setting; and multiparous are at risk of contracting hepatitis B infection (6). However, many of them demonstrated positive attitudes toward receiving the HB vaccine. In fact, many of them would like to get their baby protected against HB viral infection, to the extent that they are ready to allow their baby take anti-HBV antibodies and/or also take drugs, themselves, to prevent the transmission of HBV to their baby, if infected with HBV. This shows that the respondents were very receptive to getting vaccinated against HBV.

However, this study has its limitations. First of all, this study did not objectively determine the HB sero-positivity and vaccination status of the respondents. Secondly, this study is a hospital-based study; only those that presented at the antenatal clinics of the surveyed public hospitals were recruited for the study. Based on the limitations and findings made in this study, authors would like to suggest the following:

- Conduction of a big community-based study among pregnant women in the various communities situated within Sokoto City, Nigeria. This kind of study will be able to cover the population of women who do not visit antenatal clinics during pregnancy.
- Proper education of pregnant women and their spouses on MTCT of HBV as well as the benefits of HB vaccination.
- More efforts need to be put by local and international governmental and non-governmental in supporting the HBV vaccination programs in Nigeria, so that Nigeria can achieve her set goal of eradicating MTCT of HBV.

Conclusion

The findings made from this study had established that there is a very low awareness rate on hepatitis B vaccine amongst pregnant women in Sokoto City, Nigeria; however, many of them would be glad to get themselves and their babies protected against HB infection through the vaccine.

Acknowledgments

Authors have no competing interest to declare. This study was self-funded. Also, this chapter was a revised version of an earlier publication of the authors (27).

REFERENCES

[1] Hwang EW, Cheung R. Global epidemiology of hepatitis B virus (HBV) infection. N Am J Med Sci (Boston) 2011;4(1):7-13.

[2] Eke CB, Ogbodo SO, Ukoha OM, Ibekwe RC, Asinobi IN, Ikefuna AN, et al. Seroprevalence and risk factors of hepatitis B virus infection among adolescents in Enugu, Nigeria. J Trop Paediatr 2015;61(6):407-13. doi: 10.1093/tropej/fmv035.

[3] Yazigi N, Balistreri WF. Viral hepatitis. In: Kliegman RM, Behrman RE, Jenson HB, Stanton BF, eds. Nelson textbook of pediatrics, 18th ed. Philadelphia, PA: Saunders, 2007.

[4] Eke CB, Onyire NB, Amadi OF. Prevention of mother to child transmission of hepatitis B virus infection in Nigeria: A call to action. Niger J Paediatr 2016; 43(3):201-8.

[5] Musa BM, Bussell S, Borodo MM, Samaila AA, Femi OL. Prevalence of hepatitis B virus infection in Nigeria, 2000-2013: A systematic review and meta-analysis. Nig J Clin Pract 2015;18(2):163-72.

[6] Anaedobe CG, Fowotade A, Omoruyi CE, Bakare RA. Prevalence, socio-demographic features and risk factors of hepatitis B virus infection among pregnant women in Southwestern Nigeria. Pan Afr Med J 2015;20:406. doi: 10.11604/pamj.2015.20.406.6206.

[7] Sodipo OY, Ebenso B. An appraisal of the prevention of mother-to-child transmission of hepatitis B virus health system in Nigeria. J Public Health Epidemiol 2017;9(12):309-17.

[8] Ikobah J, Okpara H, Elemi I, Ogapere Y, Udoh E, Ekanem E. The prevalence of hepatitis B virus infection in Nigerian children prior to vaccine introduction into the National Programme on Immunization schedule. Pan Afr Med J 2016;23:128. doi: 10.11604/pamj.2016.23.128.8756.

[9] Shepard CW, Simard EP, Finelli L, Fiore AE, Bell BP. Hepatitis B virus infection: Epidemiology and vaccination. Epidemiol Rev 2006;28:112-25.

[10] Odusanya OO. Hepatitis B virus vaccine: The Nigerian story. IFEMED J 2008;14(1):4-5.

[11] Odusanya OO, Alufohai E, Meurice FP, Ahonkhai VI. Five-year post-vaccination efficacy of hepatitis B vaccine in rural Nigeria. Hum Vaccines 2011;7(6):625-9.

[12] Odusanya OO, Alufohai EF, Meurice FP, Ahonkhai VI. Determinants of vaccination coverage in rural Nigeria. BMC Public Health 2008;8:381. doi: 10.1186/1471-2458-8-381.

[13] Breakwell L, Tevi-Benissan C, Childs L, Mihigo R, Tohme R. The status of hepatitis B control in the African region. Pan Afr Med J 2017;27(Suppl 3):17. doi: 10.11604/pamj.supp.2017.27.3.11981.

[14] Ogunlade OL. Perspectives on hepatitis B vaccination among health care workers in Nigeria. Int J Trop Dis Health. 2016;18(3):1-11. doi: 10.9734/IJTDH/2016/27450.

[15] Hassan M, Awosan KJ, Nasir S, Tunau K, Burodo A, Yakubu A, et al. Knowledge, risk perception and hepatitis B vaccination status of healthcare workers in Usmanu Danfodiyo University Teaching Hospital, Sokoto, Nigeria. J Public Health Epidemiol 2016;8(4):53-9.

[16] Adekanle O, Ndububa DA, Olowookere SA, Ijarotimi O, Ijadunola KT. Knowledge of hepatitis B virus infection, immunization with hepatitis B vaccine, risk perception, and challenges to control hepatitis among hospital workers in a Nigerian tertiary hospital. Hepatitis Res Treat 2015(2015):439867. doi:10.1155/2015/439867.

[17] Abiola AO, Agunbiade AB, Badmos KB, Lesi AO, Lawal AO, Alli QO. Prevalence of HBsAg, knowledge, and vaccination practice against viral hepatitis B infection among doctors and nurses in a secondary health care facility in Lagos state, South-western Nigeria. Pan Afr Med J 2016;23:160. doi: 10.11604/pamj.2016.23.160.8710.

[18] Ogundele OA, Fehintola FO, Adegoke AI, Olorunsola A, Omotosho OS, Odia B. Perceived risk, willingness for vaccination and uptake of hepatitis B vaccine among health care workers of a specialist hospital in Nigeria. Public Health Res 2017;7(4):100-5.

[19] Fatusi AO, Fatusi OA, Esimai AO, Onayade AA, Ojo OS. Acceptance of hepatitis B vaccine by workers in a Nigerian teaching hospital. East Afr Med J 2000;77(11):608-12.

[20] Ochu CL, Beynon CM. Hepatitis B vaccination coverage, knowledge and sociodemographic determinants of uptake in high risk public safety workers in Kaduna State, Nigeria: a cross sectional survey. BMJ Open 2017;7:e015845. doi: 10.1136/bmjopen-2017-015845.

[21] Ibekwe RC, Ibeziako N. Hepatitis B vaccination status among health workers in Enugu, Nigeria. Niger J Clin Pract 2006;9(1):7-10.

[22] Daboer JC, Chingle MP, Banwat ME. Knowledge, risk perception and vaccination against hepatitis B infection by primary healthcare workers in Jos, North Central Nigeria. Niger Health J 2010;10(1-2):9-13.

[23] Ekpenyong MS, Tawari-Ikeh EP, Ekpenyong AS. Investigation on the awareness of hepatitis B virus among health care workers in Nigeria. Nurs Palliat Care 2016;1(5):124-9.

[24] Noreen N, Kumar R, Shaikh BT. Knowledge about hepatitis B vaccination among women of childbearing age: a cross-sectional study from a rural district of Punjab, Pakistan. East Mediterr Health J 2015;21(2):129-33.

[25] Abdulai MA, Baiden F, Adjei G, Owusu-Agyei S. Low level of hepatitis B knowledge and awareness among pregnant women in the Kintampo North municipality: implications for effective disease control. Ghana Med J 2016;50(3)157-62.

[26] Jha S, Devaliya D, Bergson S, Desai S. Hepatitis B knowledge among women of childbearing age in three slums in Mumbai: a cross-sectional survey. Hepatol Med Policy 2016;1:5. DOI: 10.1186/s41124-016-0007-7.

[27] Fidelis C, Kanmodi KK, Olajolumo J. Do they actually want the vaccine? A survey on awareness and acceptance of hepatitis B vaccination among expectant mothers in Sokoto City, Nigeria. Int J Child Health Hum Dev 2019;12(2):115-20.

In: Nigeria: Perspectives of Health
Editors: Ariel Tenenbaum et al.
ISBN: 978-1-53618-090-9

Chapter 6

PREVALENCE OF SHISHA SMOKING AND AWARENESS OF HEAD AND NECK CANCER AMONG SECONDARY SCHOOL STUDENTS IN IBOKUN TOWN

Kehinde K Kanmodi[1-3,*], BDS, AISQEM, Omotayo F Fagbule[1,4,5], BDS, MWACS and Timothy O Aladelusi[1,6-8], BDS, MSc, FWACS, FAOCMF

[1]Campaign for Head and Neck Cancer Education (CHANCE) Program, Cephas Health Research Initiative Inc, Ibadan, Nigeria, [2]Department of Dental and Maxillofacial Surgery, Usmanu Danfodiyo University Teaching Hospital, Sokoto, Nigeria, [3]Community Health Officers Training Programme, Usmanu Danfodiyo University Teaching Hospital, Sokoto, Nigeria, [4]Department of Periodontology and Community Dentistry, University College Hospital, Ibadan, Nigeria, [5]Department of Community Medicine, Faculty of Public Health, University of Ibadan, Ibadan, Nigeria, [6]Department of Oral and Maxillofacial Surgery, University of Ibadan, Ibadan, Nigeria,[7]Department of Oral and Maxillofacial Surgery,

[*] Corresponding Author's Email: kanmodikehinde@yahoo.com.

University College Hospital, Ibadan, Nigeria, [8]Ninth People's Hospital, Shanghai, Peoples Republic of China

Abstract

Shisha smoking is a known risk factor for head and neck cancer (HNC). Objectives: To determine the rate of shisha smoking among secondary school students in Ibokun Town, Nigeria. Methods: This was a pilot questionnaire-based study conducted among grades 7 to 12 students in two secondary schools in Ibokun Town, Nigeria. Questionnaire obtained information from the subjects on their biodata, history of shisha smoking, awareness of HNC, and attitudes toward receiving HNC education. Results: More than half (54.0%) of the subjects were ≤14 years old, 56.6% of them were females, 97.5% were Yorubas, 50.5% were in a private school, and 82.8% were in grades 10 to 12. Only 11 (5.6%) subjects had ever smoked shisha, and 54.5% (6/11) of them were females. Only 3, out of these 11 subjects, smoked shisha for the first time at the age of 10 years or younger. Also, 7 subjects (5 females, and 2 males) reported that they smoked shisha on all the 30 days prior to their participation in the study. Lastly, less than half (47.5%) of the subjects had never heard of HNC; however, the majority (81.8%) of them showed interest in being educated on HNC. Conclusion: This study recorded a low prevalence rate of shisha smoking among the surveyed students. Many of the subjects had never heard of HNC before; however majority of them loved to be educated on HNC. Authors recommend early HNC education for secondary school students, with emphasis placed on tobacco cessation.

Introduction

Shisha smoking, according to the British Heart Foundation, is a way of smoking tobacco, sometimes mixed with fruit or molasses sugar, through a bowl hose or tube (1). Shisha smoking is also called hookah, narghile, waterpipe, or hubble bubble smoking (1, 2). Shisha smoking took its history from Asia (1, 2). In some parts of the world, shisha smoking has surpassed cigarette smoking, with its rate of use increasingly growing among children and young adults (1, 2, 3).

According to the World Health Organization, shisha smoking is an addictive behavior (2), and it has been reported that shisha smokers do take shisha in the company of relatives and friends (4-7). This reflects that shisha smoking is an acceptable social behavior in many societies.

Unlike cigarettes where their packs have warning labels about the negative health implications associated with tobacco smoking, shisha bottles do not have such warning labels (8). Shisha has tobacco as part of its constituents; hence shisha smoking is a risk factor for life-threatening diseases like cancer (2, 8). Furthermore, most of the anti-smoking policies in different nations of the world are focused on cigarette, while policies discouraging shisha smoking were not in focus (9-12). As a matter of fact, virtually no shisha-specific policy exists in many nations (2, 11, 12). In many developed countries for instance, shisha smoking venues and shisha products are exempted from tobacco control policies (9, 10).

In Nigeria, shisha is gaining its popularity and more shisha smoking venues are erected in some Nigerian discos and restaurants (2, 13). Interestingly, little or no empirical study is available on shisha smoking in Nigeria (13). This preliminary study aims to determine the prevalence of shisha smoking and also explore the awareness of head and neck cancer (HNC) among a pilot sample of school-going adolescents and young adults in Ibokun Town, Nigeria.

OUR STUDY

This preliminary study forms part of the research projects conducted during the 2016 Campaign for Head and Neck Cancer Education (CHANCE) Program (14, 15). This program was an initiative of the Cephas Health Research Initiative Inc., a non-profit indigenous non-governmental organization based in Nigeria. Permission to conduct this study was officially obtained from the authorities of the participating schools, and all subjects' participation was completely voluntary and anonymous.

Two conveniently selected secondary schools were surveyed in this study: one public school and one private school. Being a preliminary study, authors used a convenient sample of 198 students. Multistage sampling technique was used in the selection of the participating classes, while simple random sampling technique was used in the selection of the subjects from the participating classes. Prior to questionnaire administration, authors approached the students and the teachers of the selected classes in their respective classrooms; they were informed about the purpose of the study and that their participation is voluntary and confidential. Informed consent was also obtained from all that took part in the study. All questionnaires were self-administered. The questionnaire obtained information from each participant about their demographic profile, history of smoking shisha, and awareness of tobacco as a risk factor for head and neck cancer.

The collected data were cross-checked and none was discarded because they all were appropriately filled. Data was analyzed using the SPSS version 16 Software. The outcomes of the analysis were presented in tables.

FINDINGS

More than half (54.0%) of the subjects were ≤14 years old, 56.6% of them were females, 97.5% were Yorubas, 50.5% were in a private school, 82.8% were in grades 10 to 12, and 74.2% were Christians (see Table 1).

Only 11 (5.6%) subjects had ever smoked shisha, of which 54.5% (6/11) of them were females (see Table 2). Only 3, out of these 11 subjects, smoked shisha for the first time at the age of 10 years or younger (see Table 3). Also, 7 subjects (5 females, and 2 males) reported that they smoked shisha on all the 30 days prior to their participation in the study (see Table 4).Lastly, less than half (47.5%) of the subjects had never heard of HNC (see Table 5); however, the majority (81.8%) of them showed interest in being educated on HNC (See Table 6).

Table 1. Demographic profile of subjects

Characteristics (n = 198)	Frequency (%)
Gender	
Female	112 (56.6)
Male	81 (40.9)
Not specified	5 (2.5)
School grade	
Grades 7 – 9	37 (17.2)
Grades 10 – 12	161 (82.8)
Age (in years)	
≤14	107 (54.0)
15 – 18	83 (41.9)
19 – 24	3 (1.5)
Not specified	5 (2.5)
School	
Public	98 (49.5)
Private	100 (50.5)
Tribe	
Yoruba	193 (97.5)
Igbo	1 (0.5)
Others	1 (0.5)
Not specified	3 (1.5)
Religion	
Islam	47 (23.7)
Christianity	147 (74.2)
Traditional	1 (0.5)
Others	1 (0.5)
Not specified	2 (1.0)

n = Total number of the subjects.

Table 2. Comparison between gender of subjects and experimentation of waterpipe (shisha) smoking

	Response	Gender		Total	X^2 (p-value)
		Female	Male		
Have you ever tried or experimented with waterpipe smoking even one or two puffs?	Yes	6	5	11	0.521
	No	105	75	180	
Total		111	80	191	

Response	Frequency (%)
Yes	94 (47.5)
No	83 (41.9)
Not sure	11 (5.6)
No response	10 (5.1)
Total	198 (100.0)

Table 3. Comparison between gender of subjects and age at first waterpipe (shisha) smoking experience

	Response	Gender		Total	X^2 (p-value)
		Female	Male		
How old were you when you first tried smoking waterpipe (shisha)?	I have never smoked water-pipe	104	76	180	0.422
	Age 10 or younger	1	2	3	
	Age 16 to 17	1	0	1	
	Age 18 or older	0	1	1	
Total		106	79	185	

Table 4. Comparison between gender of subjects and history of recent waterpipe (shisha) smoking

	Response	Gender		Total	X^2 (p-value)
		Female	Male		
During the past 30 days, on how many days did you smoke waterpipe (shisha)?	0 day	96	71	167	0.207
	1 or 2 days	0	2	2	
	3 to 5 days	0	1	1	
	6 to 9 days	0	1	1	
	10 to 19 days	0	1	1	
	All 30 days	5	2	7	
Total		101	78	179	

Table 5. Response of subjects to the question: Have you ever heard of head and neck cancer before?

Response	Frequency (%)
Yes	94 (47.5)
No	83 (41.9)
Not sure	11 (5.6)
No response	10 (5.1)
Total	198 (100.0)

Table 6. Response of subjects to the question: Do you like to receive a comprehensive education on how to prevent head and neck cancer in future?

Response	Frequency (%)
Yes	162 (81.8)
No	30 (15.2)
No response	6 (3.0)
Total	198 (100.0)

DISCUSSION

This study surveyed a pilot sample of 198 secondary school students in Ibokun Town, Nigeria, on the prevalence of shisha smoking and awareness of HNC. In this study, we observed a very low prevalence of shisha smoking among the study subjects. Also, we found that many of the subjects had never heard of HNC and the majority of them would like to be educated on the killer disease.

Shisha smoking is an addictive behavior, also its smokes has detrimental effects on the body (2, 8). The likelihood of developing smoking habit have been reported to be very high among adolescents due to some influencing factors like peer influence, parental smoking, and poor academic performance (2, 16, 17). The age at which smoking habit is developed goes a long way in predicting an individual's level of risk of developing tobacco-associated chronic diseases; individuals with early exposure to tobacco smoking tends to have higher risk of developing such health problems when compared to those who started smoking at latter ages (18-21). It is worthy of note that some of the subjects in this study experimented shisha smoking at age 10 or younger. This suggests that some of the subjects are at risk of developing tobacco-associated chronic diseases if they continue to smoke shisha.

In this study, the lifetime prevalence of shisha use among the subjects was 5.6%. Furthermore, some few subjects were found to be active shisha smokers. Some of these few subjects smoked shisha in all the recent 30 days prior to the day of participation in the questionnaire. However, the prevalence rate of shisha smoking recorded among the subjects in this present study is very low when compared to that recorded among Pakistani and German adolescents (22, 23). The low prevalence rate recorded in this study may be because of the setting where this study was conducted, as the study area was a semi-urban area unlike the other studies which were conducted in a more developed setting.

Furthermore, we observed that the majority of the subjects had never heard of HNC. Head and neck cancer is a notorious disease which claims 300,000 lives every year (24); hence the need for public education on its risk factors, symptoms, and HNC self-examination. In this study, the majority of the subjects showed interest in getting a comprehensive education on HNC prevention. Based on their level of motivation, authors predict that the surveyed students will benefit immensely from HNC education.

However, this study has its limitations. First of all, this study can only give an estimated prevalence rate of shisha smoking among the surveyed students, because it is difficult to ascertain if all information provided by the subjects was true. Secondly, this study did not explore how and why some subjects are active shisha smokers. Hence, there is a need for qualitative study, preferably a mixed study, to explore shisha smoking habits among secondary school students in this study area. Also, this study was a preliminary survey with small sample size; authors recommend that bigger studies should be conducted on shisha smoking in Nigeria.

Conclusion

To the best of authors' knowledge, this is the first study to report shisha smoking among Nigerian adolescents. This study recorded a low prevalence rate of shisha smoking among the surveyed secondary school students in Ibokun Town. Many of the subjects had never heard of HNC before; however majority of them loved to be educated on HNC. Authors recommend that such programs should be conducted for the secondary school students in Ibokun Town.

Acknowledgements

Authors appreciate the authorities of the participating schools for approving the study. Authors also appreciate the teachers and students for their conduct during the study. This study forms part of the 2016 CHANCE Program of the Cephas Health Research Initiative Inc, Nigeria.

Authors did not receive any external funding for this research project, and they have no competing interest to declare. Lastly, this chapter was a revised version of an earlier publication of the authors (25).

REFERENCES

[1] British Heart Foundation. Shisha. URL: https://www.bhf.org.uk/heart-health/risk-factors/smoking/shisha.

[2] WHO Study Group on Tobacco Product Regulation (TobReg). Advisory note: Waterpipe tobacco smoking: health effects, research needs and recommended actions by regulators, 2nd ed. Geneva: World Health Organization; 2015.

[3] Control and prevention of waterpipe tobacco products (document FCTC/COP/6/11). Conference of the Parties to the WHO Framework Convention on Tobacco Control, Sixth session, Moscow, Russian Federation, 13 – 18 October 2014. Geneva: World Health Organization; 2014.

[4] Maziak W, Eissenberg T, Ward KD. Patterns of waterpipe use and dependence: implications for intervention development. Pharmacol Biochem Behav 2005;80:173-9.

[5] Martinasek MP, McDermott RJ, Martini L. Waterpipe (hookah) tobacco smoking among youth. Curr Probl Pediatr Adolesc Health Care 2011;41:34-57.

[6] Carroll MV, Chang J, Sidani JE, Barnett TE, Soule E, Balbach E, et al. Reigning tobacco ritual: waterpipe tobacco smoking establishment culture in the United States. Nicotine Tob Res 2014;16:1549-58.

[7] Afifi R, Khalil J, Fouad F, Hammal F, Jarallah Y, Abu Farhat H, et al. Social norms and attitudes linked to waterpipe use in Eastern Mediterranean Region. Soc Sci Med 2013;98:125-34.

[8] Bahelah R. Waterpipe tobacco labeling and packaging and World Health Organization Framework Convention on Tobacco Control (WHO FCTC): A call for action. Addiction 2014;109:333.

[9] Maziak W, Nakkash R, Bahelah R, Husseini A, Fanous N, Eissenberg T. Tobacco in the Arab world: old and new epidemics amidst policy paralysis. Health Policy Plan 2013;29:784-94.

[10] Salloum RG, Nakkash RT, Myers AE, Wood KA, Ribisl KM. Point-of-scale tobacco advertising in Beirut, Lebanon following a national advertising ban. BMC Public Health 2013;13:354.

[11] Chaloupka FJ, Straif K, Leon ME. Effectiveness of tax and price policies in tobacco control. Tob Control 2011;20:235-8.

[12] Gilmore AB, Tavakoly B, Taylor G, Reed H. Understanding tobacco industry pricing strategy and whether it undermines tobacco tax policy: the example of the UK cigarette market. Addiction 2013;108:1317-26.

[13] Global adult tobacco survey: Nigeria country report 2012. Brazzaville: World Health Organization Regional Office for Africa, 2012.

[14] Fagbule OF, Kanmodi KK, Aladelusi TO. Secondhand tobacco smoke exposure and attitudes towards tobacco ban: A pilot survey of secondary school students in Ibokun Town, Nigeria. Int J Child Adolesc Health 2018;11(3), in press.

[15] Kanmodi KK, Fagbule OF. Does head and neck cancer (HNC) education have impact on adolescents' knowledge and attitude towards HNC and HNC peer education? An example from Nigeria. Int J Child Adolesc Health 2018;11(3), in press.

[16] Kaya CA, Unalan PC. Factors associated with adolescents' smoking experience and staying tobacco free. Mental Health Fam Med 2010;7(3):145-53.

[17] Tyas SL, Pederson LL. Psychosocial factors related to adolescent smoking: a critical review. Tobacco Control 1998;7:409-20.

[18] Planas A, Clara A, Marrugat J, Pou J, Gasol A, de Moner A, et al. Age at onset of smoking is an independent risk factor in peripheral artery disease development. J Vascular Surg 2002;35(3):506-9.

[19] Flanders D, Lally CA, Zhu B, Henley J, Thun MJ. Lung cancer mortality in relation to age, duration of smoking, and daily cigarette consumption: Results from Cancer Prevention Study II. Cancer Res 2003;63(19):6556-62.

[20] Pandeya N, Williams GM, Sadhegi S, Green AC, Webb PM, Whiteman DC. Associations of duration, intensity, and quantity of smoking with adenocarcinoma and squamous cell carcinoma of the esophagus. Am J Epidemiol 2008;168(1):105-14.

[21] Will JC, Galuska DA, Ford ES, Mokdad A, Calle EE. Cigarette smoking and diabetes mellitus: evidence of a positive association from a large prospective cohort study. Int J Epidemiol 2001;30(3):540-6.

[22] Kuntz B, Lampert T, KIGGS Study Group. Waterpipe (shisha) smoking among adolescents in Germany: Results of the KIGGS Study: First follow-up (KIGGS Wave 1). Bundesgesundheitsblatt Gesundheitsforschung Gesundheitsschutz 2015;58(4-5):467-73.

[23] Anjum Q, Ahmed F, Ashfaq T. Knowledge, attitude and perception of water pipe smoking (shisha) among adolescents aged 14-19 years. J Pak Med Assoc 2008;58(6):312-7.

[24] Jemal A, Bray F, Center MM, Ferlay J, Ward E, Forman D. Global cancer statistics. CA Cancer J Clin 2011;61(2):69-90.

[25] Kanmodi KK, Fagbule OF, Aladelusi TO. Prevalence of shisha (waterpipe) smoking and awareness of head and neck cancer among Nigerian secondary school students: A preliminary survey. Int Public Health J 2018;10(2):210-4.

In: Nigeria: Perspectives of Health
Editors: Ariel Tenenbaum et al.
ISBN: 978-1-53618-090-9

Chapter 7

HEALTHCARE PROVIDER ATTITUDE TOWARDS PERSONS WITH DISABILITIES IN NIGERIA

Paul M Ajuwon[1,*], PhD, Ishiaq O Omotosho[2], PhD and Rebecca Y Stallings[3], MS

[1]Department of Counseling, Leadership and Special Education, Missouri State University, Springfield, Missouri, United States of America
[2]Department of Chemical Pathology/Clinical Biochemistry, University College Hospital, Ibadan, Nigeria
[3]Private Research Consultants, Springfield, Missouri, United States of America

ABSTRACT

In this chapter we investigate healthcare providers' attitudes towards persons with disabilities (PWDs) at the University College Hospital (UCH), Ibadan, Nigeria. The investigators utilised the Interaction with Disabled Persons (IDP) Scale to measure the attitudes of direct and

* Corresponding Author's Email: paulajuwon@missouristate.edu.

indirect healthcare providers at UCH. In all, 203 workers fully completed a questionnaire containing demographic and experiential questions and the IDP. Scores on three scale factors were analysed. The mean Discomfort score was lower for direct- versus indirect-care providers (t=-2.537; p=0.012). A higher Discomfort score was associated with a lower level of confidence in treating PWDs (r=-0.221; p=0.003). Similarly, a higher Information score was associated with lower confidence (r=-0.300; p<0.001), a lower level of training on treating PWDs (r=-0.170; p=0.018), and a lower knowledge of legislation and policies pertaining to PWDs (r=-0.180; p=0.013). The mean cubed Vulnerability score was lower for healthcare providers reporting less confidence (t=-2.201; p=0.029) and higher for older providers (t=2.073; p=0.039). Three-quarters of participants were direct-care providers, which is suggestive of physicians' willingness to deliver services to specialised populations. Recommendations are made to increase providers' confidence through in-service training, and to facilitate direct and indirect healthcare providers' organisational and individual capacities to sustain quality healthcare for PWDS.

INTRODUCTION

In numerous countries throughout the world, some factors have been identified in healthcare providers' attitudes towards persons with disabilities (PWDs). These factors, inter alia, include lack of disability-specific knowledge, discomfort with working with PWDs, fear of disability and misperceptions about disability (1-6). These challenges are so pervasive that PWDs themselves have cited poor attitudes of physicians as the most formidable obstacle to accessing healthcare services (7, 8). For the purpose of this study, we define attitudes as positive or negative dispositions towards a person, concept or situation. Our conviction is that a healthcare provider's attitude towards a patient is fundamental because existing misconceptions can potentially hinder diagnosis and treatment (9, 10).

Furthermore, a provider's disposition is particularly important when tending to patients with disabilities. This is because the healthcare professional may view an individual's disability as a negative trait, and such perception may prevent resources from effective utilizations (6, 11).

The assumption that a person with a disability has a baseline quality of life at a low threshold may lead the provider to avoid caring for the patient. Thus, adverse outcomes may be compounded and services available to patients may be limited if these subtle attitudes unduly affect the provider's actions.

PRIOR RESEARCH IN NIGERIA

A Nigerian study (3) found that more than half of 134 sampled healthcare workers noted that facilities and legislation related to the human rights of children with developmental disabilities are nonexistent in the country. In order to ameliorate the situation, the researchers advocated for inclusion of topics on developmental disorders in the curricula of nurses and allied medical practitioners.

Ayanniyi et al. (2) explored the knowledge and attitudes of 330 physiotherapists towards people with leprosy in the six geopolitical regions of Nigeria. The leprologists found that a significant number of participants exhibited fair knowledge, but poor attitudes towards leprosy. According to the investigators, the institution of training seems to influence the respondents' knowledge and attitudes. They advocated that educational and training programmes on leprosy should be emphasised at the basic training institutions for physiotherapists. Earlier, Awofeso (12) investigated the knowledge of nurses regarding leprosy, and reported that these healthcare workers not only lacked disability-specific knowledge, but also had a fear of leprosy. As a way of combatting such apprehensions, the author recommended that leprosy information be infused into the basic nursing curriculum in order to heighten awareness and minimise the stigma of leprosy throughout Nigeria.

Reis et al. (13), in the first population-based assessment of discrimination against people living with HIV/AIDS in four states in Nigeria, found that nine percent of professionals reported avoiding to care for an HIV/AIDs patient, and nine percent indicated that they had refused an HIV/AIDS patient admission to a hospital. Twelve percent of participants agreed that treatment of opportunistic infections in HIV/AIDs patients depletes resources, and eight percent indicated that treating an individual with HIV/AIDS is a waste of valuable resources. The researchers concluded that while most of the healthcare professionals reported being in compliance with ethical obligations, despite the lack of resources, discriminatory behaviour and attitudes towards patients with HIV/AIDS prevail among a significant number of healthcare professionals. They identified inadequate education and absence of treatment materials as contributing to these negative practices and attitudes.

Need for current study

The issues discussed in the preceding paragraphs attest to the need to investigate further healthcare professionals' attitudes towards PWDs in Nigeria. Nigeria is the most populous and ethnically diverse African country, comprising 182 million people (14). Using the World Health Organisation (15) disability threshold of 15% to determine the number of PWDs in the population, Nigeria now has 27,300,000 PWDs. This figure is expected to rise significantly in the future, given the increase in the causal factors of disabilities such as illnesses, road accidents, birth defects, collapsed buildings, poverty, environmental toxins, natural disasters, communal and religious conflict, lead poisoning, Boko Haram insurgency, and superstitions (16). These complex variables point to the need for each country to evaluate its own attitudes towards PWDs, since these factors are powerful, yet invisible obstacles to rehabilitation and integration. The current research was therefore conceived as a way to assess healthcare providers' dispositions towards their patients with disabilities in the country.

Our study

University College Hospital (UCH), the setting for this investigation, is strategically located in Ibadan, the largest city in West Africa. Established in 1959 as a teaching hospital to service the College of Medicine, it now has over 1,000 beds, with current occupancy rates of 55-60%, and includes 60 service and clinical departments. UCH is primarily a tertiary institution with appendages of community-based outreach. Given its location in a major urban centre and its dominant role in the country, UCH caters annually to thousands of patients with varying disabilities (17).

PROCEDURES

The research protocol was approved by the Institutional Review Boards of Missouri State University, United States and the College of Medicine, Ibadan, Nigeria. Having secured approval from the two institutions, the second author distributed a total of 500 questionnaires (described below) to workers in the hospital's 20 clinics. The distribution of the questionnaires occurred during the last quarter of 2015, and the first quarter of 2016 at monthly departmental meetings.

Two hundred and fifty completed questionnaires were returned to the secretary in the office of the second author. Thereafter, the second author mailed all completed questionnaires to the first author in the United States for data entry. All data were entered into an excel spreadsheet and imported to SPSS for analysis. In all, 203 questionnaires were found to be complete and analyzable.

Study Questionnaire

The questionnaire was prefaced by a cover letter to the participants explaining the purpose of the study and defining key terms. Disability was defined as "… an impairment in body functions that imposes limitations in activity or restricts how an individual participates in the society." Categories of disabilities were described to include those who experience orthopedic, intellectual (mental), seeing, hearing, emotional/behavioural, speaking, breathing, and other problems, including birth defects, genetic disorders and skeletal deformities. Participants were assured of confidentiality of all responses in accordance with the ethical guidelines of the two approving universities.

The questionnaire was delineated into three sections. Section one addressed basic participants' demographics, including age, gender, job title, education, and time in present position at UCH, along with experiential questions, including level of prior contact with PWDs, level of training on treating PWDS, level of confidence in treating PWDs, and knowledge of policies and legislation pertaining to PWDs in Nigeria. The second section comprised the 20-item IDP Scale developed by Gething (18). The final section of the questionnaire was open-ended, and enabled the participants to share personalised comments.

Interaction with Disabled Persons (IDP) Scale

In her 1994 paper summarising the development and validation of the IDP since its origins in 1980, Gething (19) provides the following operational definition: "The Interaction with Disabled Persons (IDP) Scale measures attitudes in terms of level of discomfort reported by nondisabled people during interaction with people with disabilities" (19). It consists of a 6-point Likert-type response scale ranging from "I agree very much," to "I disagree very much." Representative items include: "I admire the ability of a person with a disability to cope," and "It is rewarding when I am able to help a person with a disability." Individual items are scored from six for high agreement to one for high disagreement, with the exception of items 10, 14, and 15, which are intentionally reversed. A total score is computed by summing the item scores, excluding item 19, per Gething's instructions (18). A higher score is interpreted as indicating a greater degree of social discomfort in interacting with PWDs.

Gething (19) confirmed a six-factor model derived from the IDP Scale. These factors and their associated proportion of the total variance are as follows: Discomfort in Social Interaction (23.3%); Coping/Succumbing Framework (12.3%); Perceived Level of Information (6.1%); Vulnerability-1st (6.0%); Coping (5.2%); and Vulnerability-2nd (5.0%).

Statistical methods

Statistical analyses were conducted using IBM SPSS Statistics version 24. Scale and sub-scale reliabilities were assessed using Cronbach's alpha, corrected item-to-total correlations, and inter-item correlations. A cubic transformation was applied to one factor based on Tukey's Ladder of Transformation (20) to rectify a negative skew. The correlations between ordinal-level demographic and experiential variables and factor scores were assessed with Spearman's rank correlation coefficient. The differences in mean factor scores between 2-class demographic variables were assessed using the Student's t test for independent samples and Levene's test for equality of variances. For 3- or 4-level demographic or experiential variables, the overall differences in mean factor scores were assessed using the F-test from a one-way analysis of variance (ANOVA) and Levene's test for homogeneity of variances. Inter-class mean differences were further assessed using the Scheffe test for simultaneous pairwise joint comparisons, with a simultaneous type I error of 5%.

FINDINGS

Table 1 summarizes the characteristics of the study participants. Relatively small response categories were combined with adjacent categories as appropriate for this table. Two-thirds of the participants were female, and their ages ranged from 18 to 60 years. Half of participants had been in their current position from 1 to 5 years. Based on their stated job title, participants were classified as either direct- or indirect- care providers (see footnote for Table 1). Nearly 80 percent of participants were engaged in direct-care, based on this classification. Over half of participants stated that they had either daily or weekly contact with PWDs. While only 11 percent reported having received at least 40 hours of training on treating PWDs, 31 percent of participants reported having either a high or very high level of confidence in treating PWDs. One-third of participants reported that their knowledge of legislation pertaining to PWDs was either none or poor.

Table 1. Characteristics of study participants

	N	%
Gender		
Female	134	66.3
Male	68	33.7
(missing)	1	-
Age		
18-33 years	60	30.5
34-43 years	96	48.7
44-60 years	41	20.8
(missing)	6	-
Direct/indirect care provider		
Direct[a]	154	78.6
Indirect	42	21.4
(missing)	7	-
Time in present position		
1-5 years	104	52.3
6-10 years	45	22.6
11-31 or more years	50	25.1
(missing)	4	-
Prior contact with PWDs		
Daily	61	30.2
Weekly	49	24.3
At least once/month or once/3 months	31	15.3
Less frequently	61	30.2
(missing)	1	-
Training on treating PWDs		
None	64	31.8
Some	115	57.2
High (at least 40 hours)	22	10.9
(missing)	1	-
Confidence in treating PWDs		
Very low or low	25	12.3
Average	115	56.7
High or very high	63	31.0
Knowledge of legislation and policies pertaining to PWDs		
None or poor	69	34.5
Average	89	44.5
Good or very good	42	21.0
(missing)	3	-

[a] Includes physicians or surgeons, medical interns or residents, nurses, audiologists, clinical psychologists, dentists, and physiotherapists.

Abbreviations: PWDs persons with disabilities.

Interactions with Disabled Persons (IDP) Scale

A reliability analysis was performed using items comprising the total IDP Scale and coded following instructions by Gething (18, 19). Additional reliability analyses were performed using the items comprising each of the six factors identified by Gething (19). Reliability analysis for the total IDP Scale yielded a Cronbach's alpha of 0.614. It was observed that many of the corrected item-to-total correlations were very small (<0.3), and many of the inter-item correlations were negative. These observations suggest that the total IDP Scale does not form a reliable indicator for this study population. Reliability analyses for the second, fourth, and fifth factors were similarly problematic and yielded very low Cronbach's alphas of 0.180, 0.264, and 0.246, respectively. Therefore, only three factor scores were computed and retained for further analysis. Characteristics of these three factors: Discomfort in social interaction, perceived level of information and vulnerability are shown in Table 2.

A histogram of vulnerability scores revealed a moderately negatively skewed distribution. A cubic transformation was applied following Tukey (20). The univariate distribution of the cubed factor value was more symmetrical and depicted no outliers.

Table 2. Characteristics of selected IDP scale factors

Factor	N	# items	Range	Mean	Standard deviation	Cronbach's alpha
Discomfort[a]	184	6	6-30	16.15	5.54	0.70
Information[b]	195	5	5-25	13.67	4.28	0.57
Vulnerability[c]	200	2	2-12	9.65	1.91	0.57

[a] Includes items 9, 11, 12, 16, 17, and 18

[b] Includes items 3, 6, 9, 10 (reversed), and 12

[c] Includes items 4 and 5; this is Gething's second Vulnerability factor

Abbreviations: IDP Interaction with Disabled Persons.

IDP Factors by Participant Characteristics

A Spearman rank correlation coefficient was computed for each combination of the three IDP factors and each ordinal or interval level participant characteristic. These results are displayed in Table 3. Discomfort was significantly negatively correlated with the level of confidence in treating PWDs (r= -0.221). Information was negatively correlated with level of training on treating PWDs (r= -0.170), confidence (r= -0.300), and knowledge of legislation and policies pertaining to PWDs (r= -0.180).

Table 3. Spearman Rank correlation coefficients for selected IDP factors by study participants' characteristics

	Discomfort	Information	Vulnerability
Age (years)	-0.065 (0.389)	-0.139 (0.056)	0.136 (0.058)
Time in present position	0.034 (0.646)	-0.033 (0.651)	0.003 (0.969)
Prior contact with PWDs	-0.077 (0.303)	0.005 (0.948)	0.056 (0.434)
Training on treating PWDs	-0.090 (0.225)	-0.170 (0.018)	0.033 (0.649)
Confidence in treating PWDs	-0.221 (0.003)	-0.300 (<0.001)	-0.028 (0.693)
Knowledge of legislation and policies pertaining to PWDs	0.007 (0.928)	-0.180 (0.013)	0.006 (0.935)

Data expressed as r (p).

Abbreviations: IDP Interaction with Disabled Persons; PWDs persons with disabilities.

The differences in mean scores for each of the three factors by gender and direct/indirect care provider were assessed using the t-test. For all other participant characteristics, relatively small response categories were combined with adjacent categories as appropriate to form three classes. These classes are the same as those shown in Table 1. The presence of an overall difference in mean scores by characteristics with three classes was examined for each of the three factors and was assessed by the F-test from one-way ANOVA. Inter-class mean score differences were measured using the Scheffe test.

The first factor "discomfort in social interaction" differed significantly by classes of two characteristics. The t-test statistic for direct/indirect care provider was -2.537 (176 degrees of freedom-df; p=0.012). The mean (standard deviation-sd) discomfort score was 15.57 (5.22) for direct- versus 18.05 (5.64) for indirect-care providers. The F-test statistic for level of confidence in treating PWDs was 4.964 (2, 81 df; p=0.008). The mean (sd) discomfort scores for very low/low, average, and high/very high level of confidence were 19.05 (5.64), 16.31 (5.32), and 14.70 (5.55), respectively. This association was negative and nearly linear. The mean difference between classes very low/low and high/very high was statistically significant (p=0.009).

The second factor "perceived level of information" differed significantly by classes of two characteristics. The F-test statistic for level of confidence was 10.994 (2, 192 df; p<0.001). The mean (sd) Information scores were 16.28 (3.52), 14.00 (4.20) and 11.90 (4.05) for very low/low, average, and high/very high level of confidence. This association was again negative and linear. The mean differences between classes very low/low and average, very low/low and high/very high, and average and high/very high were all statistically significant (p=0.043; p<0.001; and p=0.007, respectively).

Similarly, the F-test for level of training on treating PWDs was statistically significant (F=4.557; 2, 190 df; p=0.012). The mean (sd) Information scores for none, some, and high level of training were 14.24 (3.96), 13.84 (4.42), and 11.10 (3.87), respectively. This association was negative, but not linear. The mean differences between classes none and high and some and high were statistically significant (p=0.014 and p=0.026, respectively). The F-test for a third characteristic, knowledge of legislation and policies about PWDs, approached the 0.05 level of significance (F=2.828; 2, 189 df; p=0.062). The mean (sd) Information scores were 14.57 (4.12), 13.40 (4.23), and 12.65 (4.44) for none/poor, average, and good/very good knowledge. This association was negative and nearly linear. The mean differences between classes were not significant at the 0.05 level.

The re-expressed third factor "vulnerability" differed significantly by level of confidence (F=3.049; 2, 197 df; p=0.050). The mean (sd) cubed vulnerability scores for very low/low, average, and high/very high level of confidence were 1178 (443), 942 (424), and 1021 (479), respectively. The mean vulnerability score was higher among healthcare providers who reported very low or low confidence in treating PWDS than for providers reporting a higher level of confidence. However, the mean differences between classes were not significant at the 0.05 level. The classes were recombined to compare very low/low versus average/high/very high means; a t-test was computed and was statistically significant (t=-2.201, 198 df, p=0.029).

The F-test for age group was marginally significant (F=2.363; 2, 191 df; p=0.097). The mean (sd) cubed Vulnerability scores were 991 (414), 942 (466), and 1124 (442) for age groups 18-33, 34-43, and 44-60, respectively. The mean vulnerability score was higher among the oldest healthcare providers (ages 44-60 years) than for younger providers. The mean differences between classes were not significant at the 0.05 level. The classes were recombined to compare age 18-43 versus 44-60 means; a t-test was computed and was statistically significant (t=2.073, 192 df, p=0.039).

In order to better explain the finding of a lower mean Discomfort score for workers classified as direct- versus indirect-care providers, the distributions of other participant characteristics were examined by direct/indirect care status. Direct care providers did not differ from indirect care workers by gender, age, prior contact, or knowledge of legislation/policies. However, direct-care providers had lower representation in the mid-range (6-10) of years in current position at UCH (Chi-square =7.912, 2 df, p=0.019), were more likely to report having had a high (at least 40 hours) level of training on treating PWDs (Chi-square =12.437, 2 df, p=0.002), and were less likely to report a very low or low level of confidence in treating PWDs (Chi-square =13.359, 2 df, p=0.001) as compared to indirect -care providers.

Similarly, the finding of a higher mean vulnerability score for the oldest healthcare workers (44-60) versus younger workers was explored further by examining the distributions of other participant characteristics by two age groups (18-43 versus 44-60). Older workers did not differ from younger workers by direct/indirect care status, training, confidence, or knowledge of legislation/policies. Older workers were more likely to be female (Chi-square =4.849, 1 df, p=0.028) and had lower representation in the weekly contact class for level of prior contact with PWDs (Chi-square =8.507, 3 df, p=0.037) as compared to younger workers. As expected intuitively, older workers were more likely to have been employed in their current position in the highest class of 11 or more years (Chi-square =81.803, 2 df, p<0.001) than younger workers.

DISCUSSION

In this study, healthcare workers in direct patient care positions had lower scores, on average, on the IDP factor Discomfort in Social Interactions with PWDs as compared to workers whose positions connote indirect care. We found a significant negative correspondence between the IDP factor Discomfort and confidence in treating PWDs, and between the IDP factor Information and confidence, level of training on treating PWDs, and knowledge of legislation pertaining to PWDs. Additionally, workers reporting a lower level of confidence had higher scores, on average, on the IDP factor Vulnerability-2nd than their colleagues reporting more confidence, and likewise for older versus younger workers.

The findings noted above are similar to results obtained elsewhere (1, 4, 21, 22). In California, McNeal and colleagues (4) found that majority of primary care physicians have at least some difficulty in examining patients with physical disabilities and many are uncomfortable in managing their care. Similarly, a Nepalese study by Devkota et al. (21) found provider's attitude towards pregnant women with disability to be negative with poor knowledge and skills about service provision. In a Canadian investigation, Aragon et al. (1) noted that six percent of their respondents did not think they could safely treat a patient with epilepsy, because they lacked knowledge of people living with the disability. Along the same vein, Al-Adawi et al. (22) stated that the majority of their study participants in Oman thought that people with epilepsy have more predispositions towards dysfunctional personality and behavioural characteristics than do "normal" people. They suggested that a developing country like Oman must inculcate in their physicians more realistic attitudes towards individuals with epilepsy.

Our extensive search of the literature indicates that this is the first time in Nigeria the IDP Scale has been used to measure the attitudes of practicing healthcare providers towards PWDs. Healthcare providers are likely to be among the first individuals with whom a newly disabled person has contact, so their dispositions towards PWDs can have significant implications for implementing treatment, rehabilitation, and reintegration into the community. Yet, as has been shown in our review of previous studies, the literature is generally inconclusive about the attitudes of these professionals.

Our study findings indicate that healthcare workers who provide direct patient care are more comfortable when interacting with their patients with disabilities as compared to workers providing indirect care. Direct/indirect care provider status was not associated with the experiential variables level of prior contact with PWDs and knowledge of legislation regarding PWDs in this sample, but level of training specific to PWDs and confidence in treating PWDs were. Hence, it may be that a larger amount of specialised training leads to greater confidence in treating PWDs.

We found that older (age 44-60 years) healthcare workers express more feelings of vulnerability about becoming disabled. Age was not associated with the experiential variables with the exception of level of prior contact, for which there was no uniform trend. Hence, it may be that we are simply capturing the recognition that, as one ages, the likelihood of experiencing a significant disabling condition is increasing, resulting in one's feelings of vulnerability.

The negative association that we observed between each of the three factor scores, discomfort, information and vulnerability, with level of confidence in treating PWDs provides support for the multi-dimensionality of the IDP Scale. Forlin, Fogarty and Carroll (23) preferred to label the factor Information as Uncertainty. Our findings indicate that less training specific to PWDs and less knowledge of legislation and policies result in more uncertainty in dealing with patients with disabilities.

A major take-away from this study is the need for healthcare providers to be adequately trained in disability-related topics while in residency or medical, nursing, or allied health professional training. Oredugba and Sanu (11), in their survey of dentists in Nigeria, alluded to this salient point when they commented that improved training would help the dentists better manage patient behaviour and utilise time effectively. Given the pervasive nature of disabilities in the Nigerian society today, proactive measures should be embarked upon so healthcare practitioners are sufficiently prepared to deal with existing and emerging disabling conditions (16). We believe healthcare providers' attitudes can influence their behaviour towards their patients. Therefore, it is critical periodically to examine their attitudes towards their patients with disabilities who come to the hospital for treatment and care.

Recommendations

From the insights gained in this study, we recommend a number of measures to develop and sustain practitioners' attitudes towards PWDs and their families. First, there should be regular in-service training sessions where healthcare providers participate in structured role-plays to experience the use of the wheelchair around the premises, wearing ear plugs and using a blindfold with a human guide to simulate walking difficulty, deafness and blindness, respectively. Second, hospital management and staff could collaborate with the Joint National Association of Persons with Disabilities, an umbrella organisation of PWDs in Nigeria, to recruit competent guest speakers with disabilities and their families to share their experiences during in-service training sessions. Third, hospital management could organise healthcare providers' visits to special education schools and rehabilitation centres for PWDs to gain authentic insights into issues that impact the special populations.

Surveys at participating institutions before and after such educational interventions (including a scale such as the IDP) could be conducted to assess changes in attitudes towards persons with disability. Further and ongoing research on the attitudes, knowledge and practices of the providers would also help to determine, over a sustained period, if health-related government policies are being implemented to promote inclusive, quality healthcare for all PWDs.

Limitations of the study

Because data for this project were gathered from one hospital, the nature of the sample limits the generalisability of the results. Therefore, we recommend expanded investigations to include selected hospitals in the six geopolitical regions of the country, including the Federal Capital Territory, Abuja. This would enable the researchers to capture responses from healthcare providers with a wider range of exposure to, and experience with, individuals with disabilities. This could result in a sample for which the total IDP Scale would prove to be a reliable indicator, as was shown for healthcare providers in other countries (24).

CONCLUSION

One notable aspect of our study is that three-quarters of participants were direct care providers, which is suggestive of the willingness of workers at UCH to implement specialized services. Significantly, over half of respondents indicated they had either daily or weekly interactions with patients with disabilities. However, only 11% reported having acquired at least 40 hours of disability-related training, and only 31% stated having either a high or very high level of confidence in treating PWDs. As members of the caring profession, direct- and indirect- healthcare providers have critical roles to play in the provision of quality health services. Therefore, it will behoove providers to be cognizant of the needs, wants and choices of PWDs. Furthermore, these healthcare providers must engage in frequent contact with PWDs in order to develop providers' confidence and foster organisational and individual capacities that will empower PWDs to live fully inclusive lives in their communities.

ACKNOWLEDGMENTS

The authors declare no conflict of interests. No potential conflict of interest was reported by the authors. There was no research funding for this study, and no restrictions have been imposed on free access to, or publication of, the research data.

REFERENCES

[1] Aragon CE, Hess T, Burneo GG. Knowledge and attitudes about epilepsy: A survey of dentists in London, Ontario. J Can Dent Assoc 2009;75(6):450a-g.

[2] Ayanniyi O, Duncan FO, Adeniyi AF. Leprosy: Knowledge and attitudes of physiotherapists in Nigeria. Disabil CBR Inclusive Dev 2013;24(1):41-55.

[3] Bakare MO, Ebigbo PO, Agomoh AO, Eaton J, Onyeama GM, Okonkwo, KO, et al. Knowledge about childhood autism and opinion amongst healthcare workers on availability of facilities and law caring for the needs and rights of children with childhood autism and other developmental disorders in Nigeria. BMC Pediatr 2009;9:12. doi: 10.1186/1471-2431-9-12.

[4] McNeal L, Carrothers LA, Premo B. Providing primary health care for people with physical disabilities: A survey of California physicians. Pomona, CA: Center Disability Issues Health Professions, 2002.

[5] Roush S. Health professionals as contributors to attitudes towards persons with disabilities. A special communication. Phys Ther 1986;66(10):1551-4.

[6] Division for Social Policy and Development. Convention on the Rights of Persons with Disabilities [Internet]. United Nations; 2006. URL: https://www.un.org/development/desa/disabilities/convention-on-the-rights-of-persons-with-disabilities/convention-on-the-rights-of-persons-with-disabilities-2.html.

[7] Harmer L. Health care delivery and deaf people: Practice, problems and recommendations for change. J Deaf Stud Deaf Educ 1991;4(2):73-110.

[8] Kinsler JJ, Wong MD, Sayles JN, Davis C, Cunningham WE. The effect of perceived stigma from a health care provider on access to care among a low-income HIV-positive population. AIDS Patient Care STDs 2007;21(8):584-92.

[9] Khan AM, Umar M, Naeem A, Marryam, M. Attitudes of medical professionals towards persons with disabilities. Ann Pak Inst Med Sci 2016;12(1):17-20.

[10] Paris MJ. Attitudes of medical students and health-care professionals towards people with disabilities. Arch Phys Med Rehabil 1993;74(8):818-25.

[11] Oredugba FA, Sanu OO. Knowledge and behaviour of Nigerian dentists concerning the treatment of children with special needs. BMC Oral Health 2006;6:9. doi:10.1186/1472-6831-6-9.

[12] Awofeso N. Appraisal of the knowledge and attitudes of Nigerian nurses towards leprosy. Lepr Rev 1992;63(2):169-72.

[13] Reis C, Heisler M, Amowitz LL, Moreland RS, Mafeni JO, Anyamele C, Lacopino V. Discriminatory attitudes and practices by health workers towards patients with HIV/AIDS in Nigeria. PLoS Med 2005;2(8):e246. doi:10.1371/journal.pmed.0020246.

[14] Nigeria. National Population Commission. Nigeria's population now 182 million [Internet]. URL: http://population.gov.ng/nigerias-population-now-182-million-npc/.

[15] World Health Organisation. World report on disability [Internet]. Geneva: WHO, 2011. URL: http://www.who.int/disabilities/world_report/2011/en/.

[16] Ajuwon PM, Lesi FEA, Odukoya O, Melia C. Attitudes of medical students towards disabilities in Nigeria. Int J Disabil Hum Dev 2015;14(2):131-40.

[17] College of Medicine. University of Ibadan. URL: https://www.com.ui.edu.ng/index.php/en/about.

[18] Gething L. Interaction with Disabled persons: Manual and kit. Sydney: University of Sydney, 1991.

[19] Gething L. The Interaction with Disabled Persons Scale. J Soc Behav Pers 1994;9(5):23-42.

[20] Tukey JW. Exploratory data analysis. Reading, MA: Addison-Wesley, 1977.

[21] Devkota HR, Murray E, Kett M, Groce N. Healthcare provider's attitude towards disability and experience of women with disabilities in the use of maternal healthcare service in rural Nepal. Reprod Health 2017;14(1):79. doi: 10.1186/s12978-017-0330-5.

[22] Al-Adawi S, Al-Ismaily S, Martin R, Al-Naamani A, Al-Riyamy K, Al-Maskari M, et al. Psychosocial aspects of epilepsy in Oman: Attitude of health personnel. Epilepsy 2001;42(11):1473-81.

[23] Forlin C, Fogarty G, Carroll A. Validation of the factor structure of the Interactions with Disabled Persons Scale. Aust J Psychol 1999;1(51):50–5.

[24] Gething L. Nurse practitioners' and students' attitudes towards people with disabilities. Aust J Adv Nurs 1992;9(3):25-30.

In: Nigeria: Perspectives of Health
Editors: Ariel Tenenbaum et al.
ISBN: 978-1-53618-090-9

Chapter 8

FACTORS INFLUENCING THE CHOICE OF GRADUATING MEDICS IN PURSUING A MEDICAL CAREER WITH THE NIGERIA DEFENCE FORCES

Kehinde K Kanmodi[1-3,*], BDS,
Ismail O Adesina[1-4], MBBS
and Abass A Moshood[1-4], MBBS
[1]Cephas Health Research Initiative Inc, Sokoto, Nigeria
[2]Community Health Officers Training Programme,
Usmanu Danfodiyo University Teaching Hospital, Sokoto, Nigeria
[3]Department of Dental and Maxillofacial Surgery,
Usmanu Danfodiyo University Teaching Hospital, Sokoto, Nigeria
[4]Department of Internal Medicine, Usmanu Danfodiyo University
Teaching Hospital, Sokoto, Nigeria

* Correspondening Author's Email: kehindekanmodi@gmail.com.

Abstract

In this chapter we explore the interest of graduating medical students in the Usmanu Danfodiyo University (UDU), Sokoto, Nigeria, on taking up medical jobs in the Nigeria defence sector. Methods: This study was a cross-sectional questionnaire survey of 63 graduating medical students of UDU, Sokoto, Nigeria. Collected data was analysed using the SPSS version 16 software. Results: The mean (±SD) age of the 63 respondents was 24.87 (±2.17) years, and the majority (73.0%) of them were males. Only 26 (41.3%) out of the 63 respondents showed interest in taking up a medical job position in the Nigeria defence sector, and the majority (22/26, 84.6%) of them were men. The majority (57.7%) of those respondents who desired working in this sector would like to work with the Nigeria Armed Forces (NAF), and their most desired arm of the NAF was the Nigeria Navy. Personal interest (65.4%), prestige (57.7%), and job security/advancement prospects (38.5%) were the top three motivating factors among those respondents that desired a medical job in the Nigeria defence sector. Conclusions: This study shows that only the minority of the surveyed graduating medics would like to take up a medical job position in the Nigeria defence sector. Personal interest, prestige, and job security/advancement prospects were the predominant motivating factors among those that desired medical job positions in the Nigeria defence sector.

Introduction

There are diverse career paths to choose from after bagging a degree in human medicine. The work of a medical doctor goes beyond clinical and as a matter of fact, a medical doctor can also work as an administrator, a policy maker, an educator, or a scientist. For instance, if we focus on the Nigeria defence sector, we will observe that the services of medical doctors are seriously needed in the Nigerian defence sector. Some of the roles played by medical doctors in the establishments under the Nigeria defence sector includes provision of medical care to defence personnel and their family, provision of medical care to civilians at warring places and other conflict zones home and abroad, planning and execution of emergency medical care and services to victims of natural disasters, amidst other duties.

Globally, career choice of medical students in the defence sector had been sparsely reported. However, from the few studies available, it was found that career in the defence sector was very appealing to medical students in Pakistan and the United States of America (1, 2), and many factors had been documented to influence the career choice of these students in the defence sector. Some of these factors include national patriotism, high income, and attractiveness of the uniform (1, 2). However, to the best of the authors' knowledge, no literature had particularly explored Nigerian medical students' choice of career with the Nigeria defence sector. Hence, authors aim to conduct this study to determine the level of interest of the graduating medics of the Usmanu Danfodiyo University (UDU), Sokoto, Nigeria, in pursuing a medical career in the Nigeria defence sector, and to also explore the factors that influence their career choice in this sector.

OUR STUDY

This research was a cross-sectional study conducted among the final year medical students of the UDU, under the ethical guidelines of the Helsinki Declaration. This institution is a public university situated within the metropolitan city of Sokoto, Nigeria. The instrument adopted for the study was a well-structured 27-item questionnaire developed through review of literatures (1, 3). The questionnaire obtained information on the bio-data, interest of participants in taking up medical jobs in the defence sector, and the factors that influenced their choice of career in these job positions.

The study population comprises 98 graduating medical students. These students were approached at their classroom and dormitories. The aims and objectives of the study were clearly explained to them before obtaining verbal informed consents for participation. However, only 63 students volunteered to participate in this study. For the sake of confidentiality, an anonymous questionnaire was used for data collection. Data collection was done in November, 2017. Collected data was entered into the SPSS version 16 software for analysis. Frequency distributions of all variables were determined, and comparisons between qualitative variables was done using Chi-square with the level of significance set to a p-value<0.05.

Table 1. Demographic profile of respondents

Attributes (n=63)	Frequency (%)
Mean age in years (±SD)	24.87 (±2.17)
Gender	
Male	46 (73.0)
Female	17 (27.0)

n=Total number of respondents.

Table 2. Comparison between gender of respondents and their interest of taking up a medical job in the Nigeria defence sector

		Gender		Total (N=63)	
		Male (N=46)	Female (N=17)		X^2
Can you take up a medical job in the Nigeria defence sector?	Yes	22 (47.8)	4 (23.5)	26 (41.3)	0.173, df=2
	No	16 (34.8)	10 (58.8)	26 (41.3)	
	Yet to decide	8 (17.4)	3 (17.6)	11 (17.5)	
	Total	46 (100.0)	17 (100.0)	63 (100.0)	

FINDINGS

The mean (±SD) age of the respondents was 24.87 (±2.17) years. Gender distribution of the respondents was skewed with the majority (73.0%) of them being males (see Table 1). Only 26 (41.3%) out of the 63 respondents showed interest in taking up a medical job in the Nigeria defence sector, of which the majority (84.6%) of them (i.e., those who desired a career in the Nigeria defence sector) were men (see Table 2).

The majority (57.7%) of those respondents who desired working in the Nigeria defence sector would like to work in the Nigeria Armed Forces (NAF), and the most desired arm of the NAF was the Nigeria Navy (see Figure 1). Personal interest (65.4%), prestige (57.7%), and job security/advancement prospects (38.5%) were the top three motivating factors among those respondents that desired a medical job in the Nigeria defence sector (see Table 3).

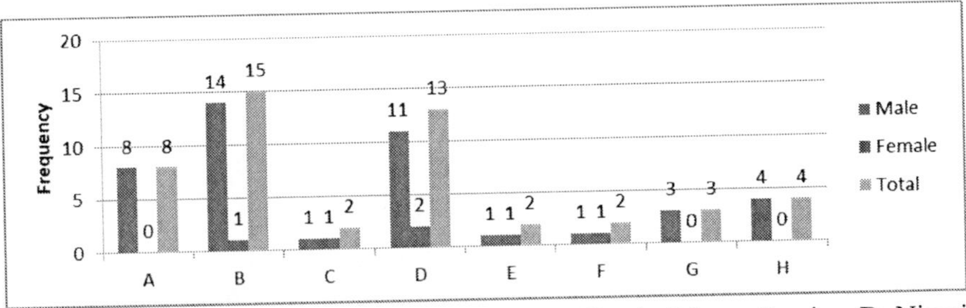

Keywords: A=Nigeria Army; B=Nigeria Navy; C=Nigeria Prisons Service; D=Nigeria Air Force; E=Nigeria Police Force; F=Nigeria Security and Civil Defence Corps; G=Nigeria Customs Service; H=National Drug Law Enforcement Agency.

Figure 1. Places where those respondents who showed interest in working with the Nigeria defence forces desired (N=26).

Table 3. Factors influencing the career choice of those respondents that showed interest in taking up a medical job position in the Nigeria defence sector

Influencing factors	Gender*		Total (N=26)
	Male (N=22)	Female (N=4)	
Personal interest	16 (72.7)	1 (25.0)	17 (65.4)
Job security/advancement prospects	8 (36.3)	2 (50.0)	10 (38.5)
Lifestyle and the job description	9 (40.9)	0 (0.0)	9 (34.6)
Prestige	13 (59.1)	2 (50.0)	15 (57.7)
Flexibility of the profession	3 (13.6)	0 (0.0)	3 (11.5)
High wages	6 (27.3)	1 (25.5)	7 (26.9)
Easily compatible with having a family	5 (22.7)	1 (25.5)	6 (23.1)
Influence from a mentor	7 (31.8)	1 (25.5)	8 (30.8)
Enough time for leisure activity	3 (13.6)	0 (0.0)	3 (11.5)
Influence from a family or relative	3 (13.6)	1 (25.5)	4 (15.4)
Gender distribution in the job	6 (27.3)	1 (25.5)	7 (26.9)

N=Total number of respondents in each category.

Discussion

Doctors-in-training in foreign countries like Pakistan and United States of America had been reported to show keen interest in taking up medical job positions with their homeland defence forces, after graduation from medical school (1, 2); national patriotism, high income, and attraction for uniform, were the predominant motivating factors that were found to have influenced their choice of career with the defence forces of their country (1, 2). Interestingly, to the best of the authors' knowledge, no similar study is available from a similar study population in Nigeria. The rationale for conducting this present study was to provide the first literature that explores Nigerian medical students' choice of medical career with the Nigerian defence forces.

In this study, it was observed that less than half of the respondents would like to take up a medical job position in the Nigerian defence sector (see Table 1). Most of those respondents that showed positive interest in working in the Nigerian defence sector preferred to work within the arms of the NAF (i.e., the Nigeria Army, Nigeria Navy, and Nigeria Air Force); this may be because the NAF is the most prestigious and powerful arm of the defence sector of Nigeria.

Interestingly, none of the female respondents in this present study would like to take up a medical career with the Nigerian Army, Nigerian Customs Service, and the National Drug Law Enforcement Agency. Unfortunately, the precise reasons why the female folks showed no interest in this study were not given in the scope of this study. However, this finding has generated research questions that need to be answered through further studies.

It is also noteworthy that the factors that informed the respondents' choice of career with the Nigeria defence forces are diverse and numerous. The top three influencing factors, among all, were personal interest, prestige, and job security/advancement prospects; interestingly, these top three factors were put into consideration by both genders. However, we observed that there were some other motivating factors that were not put into consideration by both genders. For instance, factors like job flexibility, lifestyle and job description, and enough time for leisure activities were not considered by any of the female respondents; this finding is dissimilar with other existing studies on career choice among Nigerian students in clinical professions (3, 4), as the females in those studies considered these aforementioned factors.

Our findings have its implications. First of all, the majority of the surveyed medical students had no interest in working with the Nigeria defence forces; this may pose a problem to the holistic healthcare of the Nigerian security personnel if similar disinterest is recorded among medical students in other Nigerian medical schools. There also exists skewed distribution in the choices of the medical students, as many of them preferred to work in the Nigeria Armed Forces, while a scanty few would like to work in the paramilitary and police forces. This shows that some security agencies/forces may find it very difficult to recruit medical personnel into their setting as such agencies are not appealing to medical students, as demonstrated in this study.

Lastly, this study has its limitations. Firstly, this study did not enquire into reasons why the respondents showed no interest in medical careers in the Nigeria defence sector. Secondly, this study was a single centre study and it did not survey other graduating medics in other Nigerian medical schools; hence the need for multi-centre studies that will capture a larger population.

Conclusion

This study shows that many medical students would not want to take up a medical job positions in the Nigerian defence sector. However, the majority of those that would like to work in this sector preferred the NAF. Motivating factors like personal interest, prestige, and job security/advancement prospects were the most predominant factors that were found to influence medical students' decision in taking up a medical job positions in the Nigeria defence sector.

Acknowledgments

This study is self-funded. Authors have no competing interest to declare. Also, this chapter was a revised version of an earlier publication of the authors (5).

References

[1] Attaur-Rasool S, Hasan S, Bhatti A. Early career intentions of newly inducted medical students in a private medical college in Pakistan. Gomal J Med Sci 2015;13(4):211-6.

[2] DeZee KJ, Byars LA, Magee CD, Rickards G, Durning SJ, Maurer D. The ROAD confirmed: Ratings of specialties' lifestyles by fourth-year US medical students with a military service obligation. Fam Med 2013; 45(4):240-6.

[3] Kanmodi KK, Badru AI, Akinloye AG, Wegscheider WA. Specialty choice among dental students in Ibadan, Nigeria. Afr J Health Professions Educ 2017;9(1):21-3.

[4] Oku OO, Oku AO, Edentekhe T, Kalu Q, Edem BE. Specialty choices among graduating medical students in University of Calabar, Nigeria: Implications for anesthesia practice. Ain-Shams J Anesthesiol 2014;7(4):485-90.

[5] Kanmodi KK, Adesina IO, Moshood AA. Factors influencing the choice of graduating medics in pursuing a medical career with the Nigeria defence forces: A survey. Int Public Health J 2019;11(2):117-21.

In: Nigeria: Perspectives of Health
Editors: Ariel Tenenbaum et al.
ISBN: 978-1-53618-090-9

Chapter 9

AFTER MEDICAL SCHOOL, WHAT NEXT?

Kehinde K Kanmodi[1,2,3,*], BDS, Abass A Moshood[1,4], MBBS and Ismail O Adesina[1,4], MBBS

[1]Cephas Health Research Initiative Inc, Sokoto, Nigeria, [2]Community Health Officers Training Programme, Usmanu Danfodiyo University Teaching Hospital, Sokoto, Nigeria, [3]Department of Dental and Maxillofacial Surgery, Usmanu Danfodiyo University Teaching Hospital, Sokoto, Nigeria, [4]Department of Internal Medicine, Usmanu Danfodiyo University Teaching Hospital, Sokoto, Nigeria

ABSTRACT

Not all medical students want to further their education after bagging a medical degree. Even among those who want to further, not all of them want to pursue postgraduate disciplines in clinical medicine. This study aims to explore the postgraduate disciplines desired by the graduating medical students of the Usmanu Danfodiyo University (UDU), Sokoto, Nigeria, and also explore the factors that influenced their choice of a postgraduate study program. Methods: This study surveyed a cross

[*] Corresponding Author's Email: kehindekanmodi@gmail.com.

section of 63 graduating medical students of the UDU using a well-structured anonymous questionnaire. Data obtained was analyzed using the SPSS version 16 software. Results: The mean age (±SD) of the 63 respondents was 24.87 (±2.17) years, with the majority (73.0%) of them being males. Only 44 (69.8%), out of a total of 63, respondents desired to go for postgraduate studies after finishing medical school, of which the majority (89.2%) of them desired to pursue a medical residency program. Also, not up to half (39.5%) of those respondents who desired postgraduate study intended to have it done in an institution within Africa. The disciplines chosen by those respondents who desired postgraduate studies were diverse, however the majority (70.5%) of them prefer postgraduate programs in clinical sciences. Personal interest (75.0%) and research opportunities were the top two factors influencing the respondents' choice of a postgraduate study program. Conclusions: Not all medical students desired to further their education after medical school. Also, the choices of postgraduate study programs among the surveyed students were diverse.

INTRODUCTION

After the completion of a medical degree program, a fresh medical doctor is born. As a fresh medical graduate, the next question to be asked is "What is the next task to embark upon?" Interestingly, different studies had shown that medical students have diverse preference for what to do after graduation (1-4). Those studies showed that: some medical students prefer to go into general medical practice; some prefer to pursue further educational qualifications; while some prefer to pursue other career paths that may or may not be related to medicine, after graduation (1-4).

In actual fact, there are many postgraduate disciplines that could be explored by a medical doctor, if considering further studies. As a matter of fact, specialization in disciplines within the borders of clinical sciences is just an option, amongst a gamut of options. Some of the other disciplines that could be explored include some, if not all, disciplines in social sciences, humanities, law, basic medical sciences, and public health, among others.

However, many factors had been found to influence medical students' choice of a postgraduate study program, some of which includes personal interest, ease of admission into the program, and prestige (1-4). Also, many studies had elaborately explored medical students' interest in residency training in the clinical specialties; however only scanty studies had been done on medical students' interests in disciplines outside medical sciences (1-5).

This study aims to explore the interest of graduating medical students of the Usmanu Danfodiyo University (UDU), Sokoto, Nigeria, on various postgraduate study programs, and also explore the factors that influence their choice of the proposed area of postgraduate study.

OUR STUDY

This was a cross-sectional study undertaken among graduating medical students of the Usmanu Danfodiyo University (UDU). This institution is a public university situated within the metropolitan city of Sokoto, Sokoto State, Nigeria. This institution is also the home to the only medical school within Sokoto State. A total of 98 medical students were in the graduating class during the period this study was conducted.

Study tool was a well-structured 34-item anonymous questionnaire designed by the authors through the review of literatures (1-4). Questionnaire obtained information on the: bio-data; interest of the participants in pursuing postgraduate studies after graduation; the postgraduate disciplines they would like to pursue; the continent where they would like to have the study program done; and the factors that influenced their choice of a postgraduate study program.

The participants were approached at their classroom and dormitories. The aims and objectives of the study were clearly explained to them before obtaining verbal informed consents. Only 63 students volunteered to participate in this study. Data collection was done in November, 2017.

A total of 63 questionnaires were analyzed for this study; no questionnaire was discarded because all were properly filled. Collected data was entered into the SPSS version 16 software for analysis. Frequency distributions of all variables were determined, and comparisons between qualitative variables was done using Chi-square with the level of significance set to a p-value <0.05.

FINDINGS

The mean age (±SD) of the 63 respondents was 24.87 (±2.17) years and majority (73.0%) of them were males (see Table 1).

Table 1. Demographic profile of respondents

Attributes (n = 63)	Frequency (%)
Mean age in years (±SD)	24.87 (±2.17)
Gender	
Male	46 (73.0)
Female	17 (27.0)

n = Total number of respondents.

Table 2. Comparison between gender of respondents and intention for postgraduate studies

		Gender of respondents			
Do you intend to further your education after having your medical degree?		Male (N = 46)	Female (N = 17)	Total (N = 63)	p-value (X^2), df
	Yes	37 (80.4)	7 (41.2)	44 (69.8)	0.005, df = 2
	No	5 (10.9)	8 (47.0)	13 (20.6)	
	Yet to decide	4 (8.7)	2 (11.8)	6 (9.5)	
	Total	46 (100.0)	17 (100.0)	63 (100.0)	

N = total number of respondents in each category, X^2 = Chi-square, df = degree of freedom.

Table 3. Postgraduate programs intended to be pursued by the respondents that showed interest in further studies

Postgraduate program	Male* (N = 37)	Female* (N = 7)	Total* (N = 44)
Masters	26 (70.3)	4 (57.1)	30 (68.2)
Doctorate	24 (64.9)	3 (42.9)	27 (61.4)
Residency program	33 (89.2)	5 (71.4)	38 (86.4)

*Only those that had the intention for postgraduate studies were analyzed here.

Only 44 (69.8%), out of a total of 63, respondents desired to go for postgraduate studies after finishing their undergraduate medical program (see Table 2), of which the majority (89.2%) of them desired to pursue a residency program (see Table 3). In addition, a higher proportion (80.4%) of the men, when compared to the women (41.2%) intended to further; this comparison was found to be statistically significant (p = 0.005, df = 2).

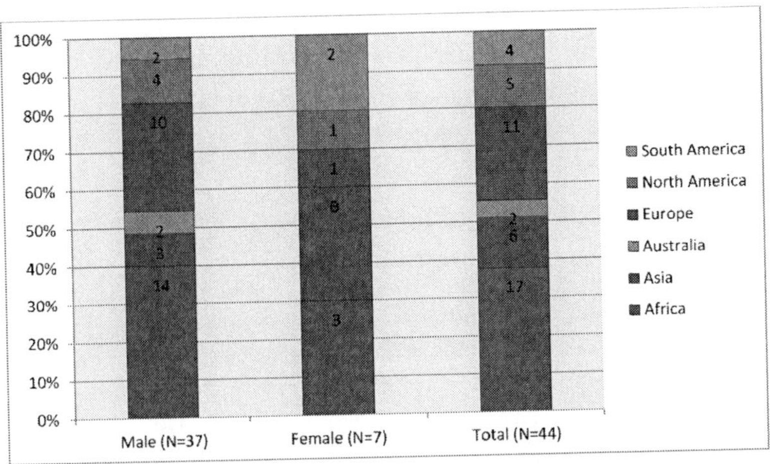

Figure 1. Continental distribution of places where respondents desired to have their postgraduate education.

Table 4. Educational disciplines desired to be pursued by those respondents that desired postgraduate education

Discipline	Gender	
	Male (N = 37)	Female (N = 7)
Social sciences	2 (5.4)	0 (0.0)
Biological sciences	1 (2.7)	0 (0.0)
Public health	20 (54.0)	7 (100.0)
Basic medical sciences	10 (27.0)	4 (57.1)
Clinical sciences	26 (70.2)	5 (71.4)
Physical sciences	3 (8.1)	0 (0.0)
Humanities	2 (5.4)	0 (0.0)
Arts	1 (2.7)	0 (0.0)
Engineering	2 (5.4)	0 (0.0)
Law	3 (8.1)	0 (0.0)

Not up to half (39.5%) of those respondents who desired postgraduate study intended to have it done in an institution within Africa (see Figure 1). Furthermore, disciplines in clinical sciences was the highest (70.5%) chosen discipline among those respondents who desired postgraduate studies (see Table 4).

Of all other influencing factors, personal interest was found to be the most popular (75.0%) influencing factor on the respondents' choice of a postgraduate study program. However, factors such as gender distribution in a study program, and other people's perception of the qualification obtained from the study program were the least popular (6.8%) influencing factors among them (see Table 5).

Table 5. Factors influencing respondents' choice of a postgraduate discipline

Influencing factors	Gender*	
	Male (N = 37)	Female (N = 7)
Personal interest in the study program	27 (73.0)	6 (85.7)
Job security/advancement prospects	14 (37.8)	1 (14.3)
Ease of entry into the study program	9 (24.3)	1 (14.3)
Lifestyle and the job description	16 (43.2)	2 (28.6)
Prestige	11 (29.7)	0 (0.0)
Opportunity to conduct research	16 (43.2)	3 (42.9)
Flexibility of the study program	8 (21.6)	3 (42.9)
Contact with patient and clinical samples	15 (40.5)	2 (28.6)
High wages	9 (24.3)	1 (14.3)
Easily compatible with having a family	9 (24.3)	2 (28.6)
Inclination of the study program before entering medical school	4 (10.8)	0 (0.0)
Influence from a mentor	9 (24.3)	2 (28.6)
Enough time for leisure activity	12 (32.4)	4 (57.1)
Influence from a family or relative	5 (13.5)	1 (14.3)
Other people's perception of the qualification obtained from the study program	3 (8.1)	0 (0.0)
Low risk of litigation	8 (21.6)	1 (14.3)
Gender distribution in the study program	3 (8.1)	0 (0.0)

N = Total number of respondents in each category, *only those that indicated interest in pursuing postgraduate studies were analyzed here.

DISCUSSION

Studies had shown that not all medical students wish to further their education after bagging a medical degree (4, 6). Furthermore, among those medical students who intended to further their education, not all of them want to go for residency training (4). In this present study, only 69.8% of the surveyed graduating medical students had the intent to further their studies, of which only 86.4% of them desired to go for residency training. This finding is lower than that reported in a previous Nigerian study, where 89.5% of the respondents in that study desired to go for residency training (7).

It is noteworthy that lack of intent to pursue a postgraduate study program was found to be more common among the female respondents when compared to their male counterparts. In fact, many female medical students do want to get married as soon as possible, after graduation, and start giving birth to children (6). Hence, the challenge of combining family responsibilities with studying may be a major reason why many of the female respondents showed no interest in postgraduate studies (8).

Furthermore, not all of the respondents considered going for postgraduate study in disciplines within medical sciences, as some of them prefer pursuing postgraduate degree programs in arts, biological sciences, engineering, law, humanities, physical sciences, public health, and social sciences. This finding corroborates with that reported among medical students in Korea (4, 5).

It is interesting to note that less than four-tenth of the study respondents who desired to pursue postgraduate studies desired to have it done in Africa. This may suggest that postgraduate qualifications from institutions domiciled in Africa are less appealing to the majority of these medical students.

The factors that influence the respondents' choice of a postgraduate study program are diverse. Personal interest was found to be the most popular influencing factors among the respondents. Similar attribute had also been demonstrated among students in other clinical disciplines (9, 10). Opportunity to conduct research, contact with patients and clinical samples, study program's flexibility, high wages, easy compatibility with having one's family, and ease of entry into a study program, were also factors that jointly influenced both the participating men and women.

We also observed that prestige, inclination of the study program before entering medical school, other peoples' perception of the qualification obtained from such study program, and gender distribution in such study program were the motivating factors that informed the women's choice of a postgraduate study program; however these factors did not inform the men's choice.

Conclusion

This study had shown that not all medical students desired to further their education after obtaining a medical degree. Among those that intended to further, not all of them want to go residency training, rather some wish to pursue degrees in fields outside medicine.

Acknowledgements

This chapter was a revised version of an article published by the authors (11).

References

[1] Alawad AAMA, Khan WS, Abdelrazig YM, Elzain YI, Khalil HO, Ahmed OBE, et al. Factors considered by undergraduate medical students when selecting specialty of their future careers. Pan Afr Med J 2015;20:102. doi: 10.11604/pamj. 2015.20.102.4715.

[2] Henderson E, Berlin A, Fuller J. Attitude of medical students towards general practice and general practitioners. Br J Gen Pract 2002;52:359-363.

[3] Morrison JM, Murray TS. Career preferences of medical students: influence of a new four-week attachment in general practice. Br J Gen Pract 1996;46(413):721-725.

[4] Kim K, Park J, Lee Y, Choi K. What is different about medical students interested in non-clinical careers? BMC Med Educ 2013;13:81.

[5] Park JH, Kim KH, Jun HR, Lee JY. A national sample survey of medical students about their perception and evaluation on medical study, career plan, and medical care system: Part 1. Survey methods and characteristics of sample. Korean J Med Educ 1999;11(2):339-363.

[6] Rabiu A, Abubakar IS, Ibrahim G, Mu'uta JI. Choice of specialization among female clinical medical students of Bayero University Kano, Nigeria. J Basic Clin Repro Sci 2017;6(1):128-133.

[7] Ossai EN, Uwakwe KA, Anyanwagu UC, Ibiok NC, Azuogu BN, Ekeke N. Specialty preference among final year medical students in medical schools of southeast Nigeria: need for career guidance.BMC Medic Educ 2016;16:259. DOI: 10.1186/s12909-016-0781-3

[8] Makama JG, Garba ES, Ameh EA. Under representation of women in surgery in Nigeria: by choice or by design. Oman Med J 2012;27:66-69.

[9] Kanmodi KK, Badru AI, Akinloye AG, Wegscheider WA. Specialty choice among dental students in Ibadan, Nigeria. Afr J Health Professions Educ 2017;9(1):21-23.

[10] Bahman RM. Career choice for nursing students in Kuwait. Greener J Epidemiol Public Health 2015;3(1):7-13.

[11] Kanmodi KK, Moshood AA, Adesina IO. After medical school; what next? A survey on graduating medical students' choice of a postgraduate study program. Int Public Health J 2018;10(2):215-9.

In: Nigeria: Perspectives of Health
Editors: Ariel Tenenbaum et al.
ISBN: 978-1-53618-090-9

Chapter 10

BARRIERS TO UPTAKE OF LOW VISION AIDS AMONG VISUALLY IMPAIRED ELDERLY NIGERIAN PATIENTS

Patrick Okonji**, OD, MPH, PhD
and Darlington Ogwezzy, OD, MBBS
Research and Innovation Office, University of Lagos, Akoka-Yaba, Lagos
and Delta State School of Health Technology, Ughelli, Delta State, Nigeria

ABSTRACT

While low vision aids enhance possibilities of reading, performing daily tasks and distant viewing for visually impaired individuals, there is paucity of research on their usage and adoption among Nigerians with low vision. Objective: This study attempts to bridge the knowledge gap about non-use of low vision aids among visually impaired older adults. Methods: Data concerning visually impaired older adults non-use of Low Vision Aids (LVAs) was collected and analysed through a cross-sectional survey in a Southwest city in Nigeria. Participants were 230 visually impaired non-users of LVAs aged 60 years and over. Results: Findings show that most non-users who were not aware of LVAs were less likely to be males, more likely to be aged over 71 years, and less likely to be middle and high educated compared to lower educated older adults. Participants aged 71 years and over were also less likely to consider future use of LVAs compared to other participants aged between 60 and 70 years. Visually impaired older adults with low levels of education were also significantly less likely to have intentions of using LVAs. Conclusion: The differences identified were mainly related to socio-demographic variables such as age, gender, household composition, and severity of vision impairment. This study highlights the importance of understanding how groups of visually impaired older adults will most likely benefit from interventions aimed at promoting uptake of LVAs and facilitating independent living among this population.

INTRODUCTION

Low vision refers to irreversible loss of vision which makes activities of daily living difficult for a person to perform (1). It is defined as visual acuity ranging from light perception to <6/18 (0.3 logMAR), or a visual field smaller than 10 degrees from the point of fixation even after treatment and/or standard refractive correction (1). However, low vision taken together with blindness represents all visual impairment (1, 2). People with low vision are, however, capable of using their residual vision and if given appropriate low vision aids and training, they do not typically need to function with additional or complementary support. In principle, many patients with low vision are not technically considered blind, although they might be classified as such. With increasing global population, the prevalence of visual impairment is increasing (2).

However, the provision and uptake of low vision services and low vision aids (LVAs) continues to be relatively low particularly in the developing countries (3, 4). In some developing countries, such as India, research focus is shifting towards identifying avenues for effective provision and uptake of low vision services (5, 6). In this context, efforts are increasingly channelled towards having data on the knowledge and awareness of low vision services among patients and eye care practitioners, and to improve quality of low vision care in the developing world (5-9).

The aim of this study was to investigate barriers to the uptake of low vision aids among visually impaired older adults in Nigeria in order to create understanding of how they can be encouraged to embrace the use of LVAs. Our focus is on older adults because it is estimated that 80 per cent of all people who need low vision care in are aged over 60 years (10). The research question explores the extent to which major barriers to accessing low vision aids hinder visually impaired older people in Nigeria from adopting LVAs. It also seeks to provide explanations on associated key factors for low uptake of low vision aids.

Low vision aids and products include a wide variety of devices designed to help those with vision disabilities live independently and make the best use of their residual vision. There are a variety of talking products that can help alleviate eye strain and improve daily living, including talking calculators, compasses, scales, cooking items, clocks, money identifiers, scales, medication reminders, talking watches, books and much more. These simple-to-use and sometimes, technology driven aids enable visually impaired individuals to take care of themselves and not have to rely on others for support. Low vision aids are frequently categorized as optical, non-optical, and electronic aids. Optical aids are useful for people with low vision as they have optical properties capable of promoting better distance and near visual performance through lenses, e.g., Telescopes (hand-held, monocular and/or binocular telescopes), High-plus spectacles (microscopes), Hand-held magnifiers, and Stand magnifiers. As optical aids require use of residual vision, they are usually more useful for individuals with low vision than for totally blind persons (11). Non-optical aids do not use magnifying lenses to improve visual function, e.g; typoscope used as a guide to reading, writing, and signature in cases of large defects of visual field, polarizing lenses used to control the reflection of light such as visors, and side shields. Electronic aids include computer and high-tech aids such as video magnifier systems, closed-circuit televisions, Bluetooth connections to smart projectors, large-print computer programs such as Zoom Text, screen readers such as Virtual Vision, Jaws, and electronic-based aids for daily living, e.g., talking clocks/wristwatches are aids with computer sound systems.

While low vision aids are essential products for low vision rehabilitation, there is scarcity of data on their use and adoption among visually impaired persons in Nigeria, as well as many developing countries. Evidence suggests that some individuals with vision impairment are, however, unaware of the myriad of low vision devices that are available and applicable to them, and others may be aware but chose not to use them (11). This is particularly a significant concern; considering that the prevalence of blindness in developing countries, is higher than developed countries. Based on figures from the Nigerian National Blindness and Visual impairment survey, it is estimated that over 2.3 million individuals suffer low vision in Nigeria (12, 13). There is a huge challenge of providing low vision services and rehabilitation for such a large population and it is important to create understanding about handy devices that can ameliorate the day-to-day challenges of living with vision impairment. In addition, the dearth of facilities and/or skilled personnels for low vision rehabilitation in Nigeria underscores the importance of interventions focusing on restoring the blind individuals' functional capacity pending other treatment alternatives. There are evidences suggesting that effective use of low vision aids promotes successful adjustment to challenges of living with vision impairment (14, 15).

In a review of existing literature regarding barriers that hinder access to low-vision (LV) care from the perspective of individuals with vision impairment, a Canadian study showed that lack of understanding about low vision services, inadequate information and miscommunication by eye care professionals, low levels of awareness about low vision care, and the need to appear independent were major barriers to accessing low vision services (16). Other factors identified by the study include negative societal views and stigma associated with use of low vision aids. However, the existence of low vision services is not synonymous to use and uptake of low vision aids. Detailed surveys in some rural communities in Nigeria have found very low uptake of public healthcare facilities despite being, in principle, within geographic proximity and free of charges (17). Understanding access to low vision services could foster knowledge, awareness, professional recommendation and use of low vision aids.

A study conducted among ophthalmologists in Nigeria cited non-availability of low vision devices within the country, lack of public awareness of low vision care, lack of training in low vision care, and practitioners (ophthalmologists' and optometrists') preoccupation with general ophthalmic practice as the major barriers in clinical low vision provision (18). Although the study focused on ophthalmologists in Nigeria, there has not been any study exploring perceptions of the end-users; i.e., the visually impaired patients, to understand the challenges of non-use from their perspective. This study therefore, attempts to bridge the knowledge gap about non-use of low vision aids from the views of intended end-users.

OUR STUDY

The study employed a cross-sectional survey method. This study adhered to the tenets of the Declaration of Helsinki and ethical approval was obtained from the Research and Ethics Committee of the School of health. Participants were aged 60 years and over. The eligibility criteria for the study included best corrected visual acuity of <6/18 in the better eye, 60 years of age and over, and the ability to read and converse in English. Participants were recruited during their routine follow-up visits in 14 registered eye clinics in the metropolitan cities of Lagos state and Delta state in Nigeria. A total of 323 visually impaired older people were contacted from 14 private eye clinics in Delta-state and Lagos state, Nigeria. The private clinics were randomly selected from five local government areas in Delta state and nine local governments in Lagos state. The study typically gathered data from surveys of views or opinions of participants as well as past clinical records of routine eye examinations. It was conducted in accordance with institutional and national guidelines for conduct of research with human subjects. The investigation was carried out in accordance with the Declaration of Helsinki of 1975 (As revised in Tokyo in 2004). Informed consent was obtained from all participants as they were briefed about the study and their verbal consent obtained before participation. Consecutive consenting respondents visiting the registered private clinics in the two states were recruited for the study. A structured interview questionnaire to ascertain socio-demographic details of participants was read out to participants and their responses recorded. Participants' low-vision case files were accessed, with their consent, to obtain relevant data on vision impairment. Of the 323 participants contacted over a period of eight months during the sampling phase of the study, 281 participants (86.99%) indicated that they did not use LVAs and were recruited to participate in the survey. However, a total of 230 participants (81.85%) participants completed the survey. Measures including: Age, gender, and vision acuity were considered as independent variables in analyses concerning non-use of LVA (see Table 1). Vision Acuity (VA) was measured using computerized Snellen chart and corresponding LogMAR values of the Snellen ratio were recorded.

Table 1. Demographic profile of participants

	N	%
Gender		
Male	92	40.00
Female	138	60.00
Age		
60-65	55	23.91
66-70	52	22.61
71-75	60	26.09
76+	63	27.39
Education		
Low	143	62.17
Medium	64	27.83
High	23	10.00
Household composition		
Single	43	18.70
Living with others	187	81.30

In the survey, participants were asked about how much they relied on others to perform daily tasks (also referred hereafter as activities of daily living). Questionnaires were printed in large fonts for partially sighted participants and read aloud for participants with severe low vision and totally blind. Appropriate boxes corresponding to their responses were ticked on the questionnaires. Dependent variables were Lack of knowledge or awareness of LVAs, Asking others for help (relying on others to perform daily living tasks), and Intended future use of LVAs. The question about Lack of awareness and Intended future use of LVAs allowed respondents to answer with yes or no. Yes was coded as 1 and no = 0. Sample questions on asking others for help included, 'I have difficulties telling the time on the clock, but I do not need a LVA because I rely on others to tell me what time of the day it is', 'I find it difficult to read, but I do not need a LVA because I rely on others to read out any printed document to me'. The question on asking others for help allowed respondents to answer on a 4-point scale: 1 (strongly agree), 2 (agree), 3 (disagree), and 4 (strongly disagree). All scores were recoded and lower scores corresponded to higher levels of reliance on others to perform tasks of daily living and therefore, not needing a LVA. Dichotomous key variables of reasons for non-use of LVAs were included. We conducted a Hierarchical logistic regression analyses using IBM SPSS statistics version 18. We initially used two-step models to investigate whether the effects of gender, education, and household composition changed with vision acuity, but as these variables did not affect the original model, we report only the final regression analysis.

FINDINGS

Among the participants, 61 percent indicated not being aware of LVAs (Mean score (M) = 0.21, and Standard Deviation (SD) = 0.41). Table 2 shows that, the non-users who were not aware of LVAs were less likely to be males, more likely to be aged over 71 years than aged between 60 and 70 years, and less likely to be middle and high educated compared to lower educated older adults. However, among this group, participants who live with others were more likely to have knowledge of LVAs than those living alone and respondents with lower vision acuity seemed to have higher knowledge and awareness of LVAs.

Table 2. Logistic regressions non-users of LVAs, alternative and future use

	Knowledge or Awareness of LVAs	Asking Others for help	Intended future use of LVAs
Constant	0.15	0.15	0.00***
Gender			
Male	0.54*	0.49*	0.78
Age (Reference: 60 – 65)			
66 - 70	0.40	0.47*	0.74
71 - 75	0.29***	0.55	0.28**
76+	0.21***	0.56	0.34**
Educational Level (Reference: Low)			
Medium	0.35	1.16	4.81***
High	0.28	1.23	4.97**
Household Composition (Ref: Single)			
Living with others	2.69**	2.65*	0.05
Vision Acuity	1.50	1.64*	4.54**
Chi-Square test	38.65***	18.94**	35.46***
Negelkerke R^2	0.15	0.001	0.29

* Significant at $p < 0.05$, ** Significant at $p < 0.01$, *** Significant at $p < 0.001$.

Approximately 58 percent of participants reported having asked someone else for help on a task requiring vision. Mean scores (M) and Standard Deviation (SD) for the variables are: M = 1.62, SD = 0.41). Men were less likely to request for help. Similarly, participants aged between 66 and 70 were more likely to request for such help compared to other age groups of visually impaired older adults. Participants living with others were significantly more likely to ask someone for help while participants with lower vision acuity were less likely to request for help. Only 23 percent of the participants indicated intentions to use LVAs in the future (M = 0.78, SD = 0.42). Participants aged 71 years and over were less likely to consider future use of LVAs compared to other participants aged between 60 and 70 years. Visually impaired older adults with low levels of education were also significantly less likely to have intentions of using LVAs. A lower visual acuity also suggested a higher likelihood of intention to use LVA in the future.

Table 3. Reasons for non-use of LVAs analysed using logistic regression

Explanatory variable	No need	Cost of LVAs	Stigma	Too old to use LVAs
Constant	7.20*	0.10	0.15	0.19
Gender (Reference: Female)				
Male	2.63*	1.02	1.03	1.15
Age (Reference: 60 – 65)				
66 - 70	0.27	1.13	10.41**	1.47
71 - 75	1.11	1.45	1.20	2.68
76+	0.96	0.86	0.60	7.68**
Educational Level (Reference: Low)				
Medium	1.16	1.39	1.21	1.13
High	0.36**	1.28	1.45	1.21
Household Composition (Ref: Single)				
Living with others	2.41*	0.98	1.43	1.56
Vision Acuity	1.17	1.19	2.13	1.35
Chi-Square test	2.42	7.67	11.17	25.62***
Negelkerke R^2	0.04	0.33	0.36	0.45

* Significant at $p < 0.05$, **Significant at $p < 0.01$, ***Significant at $p < 0.001$.

Explanations for non-use were also investigated. Table 3 shows tests of significance in differences for most important reasons for not adopting use of LVAs. The results showed that among visually impaired older adult men and women, a majority of men are more likely to not see the need for use of a LVA. Older adults aged 60-70 years were significantly more likely to report stigma as a discouraging factor for use of LVAs while older adults aged 76 years and over were significantly more likely to mention being too old to use LVAs. However, while participants with more education were significantly less likely to mention that there was ‘no need’ for LVAs, those who lived with others were significantly more likely to mention that there was no need for LVAs.

Discussion

This study set-out to investigate non-use of LVAs among visually impaired older people aged 60 years and over and important reasons for non-use. A majority of our participants reported not being aware of LVAs. This finding echoes the report from previous (and similar) studies that lack of public awareness about low vision care is a significant impediment to uptake of low vision aids and related services (4, 18). Findings suggest that, the non-users who were not aware of LVAs were less likely to be males, more likely to be aged over 71 years, and less likely to be middle and high educated compared to lower educated older adults. While findings echo a previous report that highly educated individuals are more aware of the existence of LVAs and much older participants - less technologically inclined (12), there is paucity of evidence that knowledge and awareness of LVAs is gender based. The use of LVAs might not be a male-dominated activity but stereotypically, males have been considered good with use of gadgets and historically reported as being more ICT-inclined than females (19) because women underestimate themselves in this regard (20).

Our findings also showed that a lower vision acuity was significantly related to higher knowledge or awareness of LVAs. Arguably, more severely low vision patients could be keener and more enthusiastic about exploring solutions that would remedy their sight loss in order to avoid total blindness (21). Conversely, patients with mild and moderate vision impairment are usually hopeful that their sight loss is reversible, and as such, more likely to be complacent with seeking low vision aid (4). This is further underscored in findings from this study showing that a lower visual acuity indicated a higher likelihood of intention to use LVA in the future.

Some participants reported having asked someone else for help on a task requiring vision. Findings from this study showed that when considering gender, men were less likely to request for help. This finding is consistent with previous studies showing that men are less likely to admit weakness and seek medical attention (22). It is therefore not surprising that in the investigated explanations for non-use conducted within this study, men were more likely than women to not see the need for use of a LVA.

Our participants who lived with others were more likely to report that there was no need for LVAs. This is not surprising as living with others could enhance access to alternative assistance to performing daily activities and living alone could possibly steer a compelling need for independent living aids. Similarly, participants aged between 66 and 70 years were more likely to request for help compared with other age groups of visually impaired older adults. It is possible that older participants with vision impairment have learnt ways to adapt to sight loss. As suggested by some authors, people who have lived with severely low vision for long periods are more likely to have learnt to lead independent lives than others in their early stages of mild or moderate vision impairment (23). Similarly, participants aged 71 years and over were less likely to consider future use of LVAs compared to other participants aged between 60 and 70 years. This could perhaps be so because they considered themselves too old to use LVAs and seem not to see any point in adopting use of LVAs at old ages when they have already learnt to make adjustments to cope with sight loss. Findings also showed that visually impaired older adults with low levels of education were also less likely to have intentions of using LVAs. This is not surprising given that those with higher levels of education might still see the need for use of LVAs for reading and other activities related to accessing printed materials.

From our findings, older adults aged 60-70 years were more likely to report stigma as a discouraging factor for use of LVAs while older adults aged 76 years and over did not see this as an issue. There are on-going debates that use of assistive technologies could be stigmatizing (24, 25). In some societies, social stigma still surrounds blind people due to misconceptions about blindness (16, 26). It is, however, yet to be reported that younger age groups are more cautious of the potential for stigmatising identities than older age groups. It could be argued from this aspect of the study finding that the younger age groups might be a potentially challenging group for interventions to promote adoption of LVAs among people with vision impairment. This finding adds novel understandings to the issue of social stigma and other factors impairing adoption of LVAs among visually impaired groups.

This study has some limitations. Due to the low sample size, our sample may not be fully representative of older adults' non-LVA users. Although the explored explanatory variables for non-use of LVAs among participants are moderate and consistent with previous studies of older adults' adoption of assistive technologies, it is not necessarily exhaustive. Future research should make investigate additional explanatory factors that can provide more robust explanations for visually impaired older adults' non-use of LVAs. This study investigated LVA non-use among older people in Nigeria – an emerging economy country with relatively lower availability of LVAs when compared to many first world countries. It would be insightful to replicate this study in other developing countries with similar levels of LVA and low vision services availability.

Conclusion

This study looked at visually impaired older adults' non-use of LVAs and other socio-psychological variables that may account for poor uptake of LVAs in Nigeria. The results showed that visually impaired older adults are likely to have different reasons for (dis)engagement with LVAs. The differences identified were mainly related to socio-demographic variables such as age, gender, household composition, and severity of vision impairment. This study highlights the importance of understanding how groups of visually impaired older adults will most likely benefit from interventions aimed at promoting uptake of LVAs and facilitating independent living among this population. However, more research is needed to understand attitudes of this population towards LVAs as vision impairment is not a homogenous concept and refers to a broad spectrum of needs with different levels of complexity

ACKNOWLEDGEMENTS

Conflict of interest: The authors declare that there is no conflict of interest regarding the publication of this paper.

REFERENCES

[1] World Health Organsation (WHO). Prevention of blindness and vision impairment. Refractive errors and low vision. URL: http://www.who.int/blindness/causes/priority/en/index4.html

[2] Stevens GA, White RA, Flaxman SR, Price H, Jonas JB, Keeffe J, et al. Global prevalence of vision impairment and blindness: magnitude and temporal trends, 1990–2010. Ophthalmology 2013;120(12):2377-84.

[3] Dandona R, Dandona L, Srinivas M, Giridhar P, Nutheti R, Rao GN. Planning low vision services in India: A population-based perspective. Ophthalmology 2002;109(10):1871-8.

[4] Jose J, Thomas J, Bhakat P, Krithica S. Awareness, knowledge, and barriers to low vision services among eye care practitioners. Oman J Ophthalmology 2016;9(1):37.

[5] Chiang PP, O'Connor PM, Le Mesurier RT, Keeffe JE. A global survey of low vision service provision. Ophthalmic Epidemiol 2011;18(3):109-21.

[6] Ntsoane MD, Oduntan OA. A review of factors influencing the utilization of eye care services. Afr Vision Eye Health 2010;69(4):182-92.

[7] Khan SA, Shamanna BR, Nuthethi R. Perceived barriers to the provision of low vision services among ophthalmologists in India. Indian J Ophthalmology 2005;53(1):69.

[8] Kovai V, Krishnaiah S, Shamanna BR, Thomas R, Rao GN. Barriers to accessing eye care services among visually impaired populations in rural Andhra Pradesh, South India. Indian J Ophthalmology 2007;55(5):365.

[9] Pollard TL, Simpson JA, Lamoureux EL, Keeffe JE. Barriers to accessing low vision services. Ophthalmic Physiol Optics 2003;23(4):321-7.

[10] Pascolini D, Mariotti, SP. Global estimates of visual impairment: 2010. Br J Ophthalmology 2011;96(1):11-26.

[11] Gilbert C, van Dijk K. When someone has low vision. Commun Eye Health 2012;25(77):4.

[12] Overbury O, Wittich W. Barriers to low vision rehabilitation: The Montreal Barriers Study. Invest Ophthalmology Visual Sci 2011;52(12):8933-8.

[13] World Health Organisation (WHO). Visual impairment and blindness. URL: http://www.who.int/mediacentre/factsheets/fs282/en/

[14] Bambara JK, Wadley V, Owsley C, Martin RC, Porter C, Dreer LE. Family functioning and low vision: A systematic review. J Vis Impair Blind 2009;103(3):137.

[15] Horowitz A, Brennan M, Reinhardt JP, MacMillan T. The impact of assistive device use on disability and depression among older adults with age-related vision impairments. J Gerontol Series B Psychol Sci Soc Sci 2006;61(5):S274-80.

[16] Lam N, Leat SJ. Reprint of: Barriers to accessing low-vision care: The patient's perspective. Can J Ophthalmology 2015;50:S34-9.

[17] Uneke CJ, Ezeoha AE, Ndukwe CD, Oyibo PG, Onwe F. Development of health policy and systems research in Nigeria: lessons for developing countries' evidence-based health policy making process and practice. Healthc Policy 2010;6(1):e109-26.

[18] Okoye OI, Aghaji AE, Umeh RE, Nwagbo DF, Chuku A. Barriers to the provision of clinical low-vision services among ophthalmologists in Nigeria. Vis Impair Res 2007;9(1):11-7.

[19] Margolis J, Fisher A. Unlocking the clubhouse: Women in computing. Cambridge, MA: MIT Press, 2003.

[20] Dijk van Jan AG. The network society. Social aspects of new media. Thousand Oaks, CA: Sage, 1999.

[21] Burton AE, Gibson JM, Shaw RL. How do older people with sight loss manage their general health? A qualitative study. Disabil Rehabil 2016;38(23):2277-85.

[22] Mansfield AK, Addis ME, Mahalik JR. "Why won't he go to the doctor?": The psychology of men's help seeking. Int J Men's Health 2003;2(2):93.

[23] Orr KS, Leven T. Community care and mental health services for adults with sensory impairment in Scotland. Scottish Executive Social Research, 2006. URL: http://www.scotland.gov.uk/Resource/Doc/129826/0030944.pdf

[24] Brabazon T. Beyond stigma. In: Enabling University. Springer briefs in education. Cham: Springer, 2015:61-5.

[25] Goggin G, Newell CJ. Communicating disability: What's the matter with internet studies? In 2002 ANZCA Conference, Colangatte, 2002 Jul 10-12.

[26] Beauchamp-Pryor K. Impairment, cure and identity: Where do I fit in? Disabil Soc 2011;26(1):5-17.

In: Nigeria: Perspectives of Health
Editors: Ariel Tenenbaum et al.
ISBN: 978-1-53618-090-9

Chapter 11

ATTITUDES OF A SNOWBALLED SAMPLE OF NIGERIAN HOOKAH (SHISHA) SMOKERS TOWARD TOBACCO BAN

Faruk A Mohammed[1,2], BDS, MSc,
Nwafor J Njideka[1,3], MBBS, Bashar M Aliyu[1,4], BDS,
Kehinde K Kanmodi[3,5,6,*], BDS, Dip FM, PGDE, PGDPM, PGDPSCR, CPMP, ACIPM,
Omotayo F Fagbule[3,6], BDS, MWACS, MPH
and Mike E Ogbeide[3,4], BDS

[1]Kebbi State Medical Centre, Kalgo, Nigeria
[2]Department of Oral and Maxillofacial Surgery, Jaipur Dental College, Maharaj Vinayak Global University, Jaipur, Rajastan, India
[3]Campaign for Head and Neck Cancer Education (CHANCE) Program, Cephas Health Research Initiative Inc, Ibadan, Nigeria
[4]Department of Dental and Maxillofacial Surgery, Usmanu Danfodiyo University Teaching Hospital, Sokoto, Nigeria
[5]World Health Organization Kebbi State Field Office, Birnin Kebbi, Nigeria

* Corresponding Author's Email: kanmodikehinde@yahoo.com.

[6]Mental and Oral Health Development Organization,
Birnin Kebbi, Nigeria

Abstract

Secondhand shisha smoke exposure is a cause of tobacco-induced diseases. There is a need to for the enforcement of law against shisha smoking in public places. This study aims to explore the attitudes of active shisha smokers towards the ban of shisha smoking in public places in Nigeria. Methods: A snowballed sample of 45 active shisha smokers in Birnin Kebbi was interviewed using a self-administered questionnaire. Data collected was analyzed using the SPSS version 20 software. Results: The mean (±SD) age of the surveyed active shisha smokers was 25.8 (±5.5) years, and 32 were males. Less than a third (11/45) had ever heard of the Nigeria tobacco ban law, while only a little above half were in support of tobacco ban. Conclusion: The Nigeria tobacco ban law is not popular. Despite the fact that the surveyed subjects were active shisha smokers, a majority still supported the ban of shisha smoking in public places.

Introduction

Secondhand tobacco smoke exposure is one of the major causes of tobacco-induced diseases (1-3). Unfortunately, a lot of Nigerians are exposed to these smokes (4, 5). As a matter of fact, about 14.5-55.8% of the youth living in major Nigerian cities had been exposed to this dangerous smoke in public places (4, 6, 7), making exposure to tobacco smoke an issue of public health concern in Nigeria.

In the month of May, 2015, the Federal Government of Nigeria passed the tobacco control bill into law, prohibiting smoking of tobacco in public places (such as gardens, amusement parks, schools, restaurants, healthcare centers, stadia, public transportation parks and plazas) (4). However, the enforcement of the ban was focused on cigarettes and not shisha, as more and more public shisha smoking places are being erected in the major cities in Nigeria (6-9). As a matter of fact, shisha is generally considered by the public to be a fairly harmless product, while in the actual sense shisha use is very harmful due to its tobacco content (10-14). Unfortunately, more and more people in Nigeria are now using shisha, day by day (8, 9). With the weak enforcement of tobacco ban law in Nigeria, which does not restrict the public use of shisha, many more people will continue to be active, and even passive, shisha smokers (8, 9).

Research in Nigeria had reported negative attitudes among cigarette smokers (a sub-population of smoked tobacco users) toward the Nigeria tobacco ban law (15). However, to the best of our knowledge, no published study had ever been conducted among shisha smokers in Nigeria concerning their attitudes towards this ban law. Therefore, this study aims to explore the attitudes of a sample of active shisha smokers in Birnin Kebbi metropolis, Nigeria, on the tobacco ban law in Nigeria. The significance of this study is that the outcome of this study will add new information to the body of existing knowledge on smokers' attitudes toward the tobacco ban law.

OUR SURVEY

This was a survey of 45 young active shisha smokers in Birnin Kebbi City, Kebbi State, Nigeria, which was conducted under compliance with the 1964 Helsinki Declaration on health research involving human subjects. This study forms a part of the Campaign for Head and Neck Cancer Education (CHANCE) Program organized under the aegis of the Cephas Health Research Initiative Inc, Ibadan, Nigeria (7-9, 16-17).

The sampling method and the data collection procedure used in this present study had been elaborately discussed in another article (9). Study tool was a structured anonymous questionnaire developed from a similar study (7). The questionnaire obtained information about the socio-demographic characteristics of the subjects as well as their attitudes toward tobacco ban law. Data was collected from 45 active shisha smokers. Collected data was analyzed using the SPSS version 20 software.

FINDINGS

The mean (±SD) age of the surveyed active shisha smokers was 25.8 (±5.5) years. The majority (32/45) were males, 16 had secondary school education, 27 had tertiary school education, 33 were Muslims, and 28 were from the Hausa ethnic group.

Only 11 respondents knew that there is a ban on tobacco smoking in public places in Nigeria. However, only 27 agreed that shisha sales to adolescents should be banned, 23 agreed that the advertisement of shisha and shisha products should be banned, 30 agreed that shisha smoking should be banned in restaurants, 25 agreed that shisha smoking should be banned in bars/discos/pubs, and 20 agreed that shisha smoking in all enclosed public places should be banned.

DISCUSSION

The issue of tobacco smoking in public places continues to be an issue of public health concern in Nigeria. Due to the weak enforcement of the tobacco ban law in Nigeria, many cigarette smokers in Nigeria still engage in public smoking (4-6). Due to this, more and more people have become passive tobacco smokers due to their frequent exposures to second-hand tobacco smokes (4-6). Due to the issue of weak law enforcement of the tobacco ban law in Nigeria, more and more shisha smoking places (such as discos, restaurants, hubs, etc.) had been erected in some Nigerian major cities (8, 9). Hence, this issue needs to be considered as a public health emergency.

Furthermore, the peculiarities of shisha smoking make public shisha smoking more dangerous than cigarette smoking. First, shisha is naively perceived by the many lay people, and even among its active smokers, to be a harmless product (10-14). Second, shisha smoking is widely considered as a socially acceptable behavior, unlike cigarette smoking (18-21). Third, many shisha smokers smoke shisha in enclosed public areas (such as restaurants, discos, hubs, etc.) unlike cigarette smokers, where a huge number of cigarette smokers smoke in the open air (e.g., along the street) (9). Fourth, shisha smokers often smoke shisha for a long duration, especially at social gatherings (22); hence they have the high possibility of inhaling more tobacco smokes in one sitting.

In this study, we surveyed a snowballed sample of shisha smokers on their attitudes towards banning shisha smoking in public places and interesting findings were recorded from our data analyses. We found that the majority of the surveyed shisha smokers were not aware about the tobacco ban law in Nigeria. This current finding is similar to that reported in a Nigerian study conducted among cigarette smokers by Olowookere et al. (15), where a very low awareness rate of tobacco ban was reported. This suggests the need to educate smokers, and as well the entire public on the Nigeria tobacco ban law.

However, the majority (although, averagely above half) of the shisha smokers surveyed in this study supported that shisha smoking in public places should be banned. This finding is dissimilar to that reported among a surveyed sub-population of cigarette smokers in Osun State, Southwest Nigeria, where only the minority of them were in support of tobacco ban. Nevertheless, the findings made from our study and that of Olowookere et al. (15) reveals that not all smokers (be it shisha or cigarette) are against the implementation of the tobacco ban law in Nigeria. In conclusion, the Nigeria tobacco ban law is not popular and it is also weakly enforced in Nigeria (15). Despite the fact that the surveyed subjects were active shisha smokers, majority of them still supported the ban of shisha smoking in public places.

ACKNOWLEDGMENTS

Authors have none to declare. This study was self-funded. This chapter was a revised version of an earlier publication by the authors (23).

REFERENCES

[1] World Health Organization. WHO global report on trends in prevalence of tobacco smoking. Geneva: WHO, 2015.

[2] Wang L, Mamudu HM, Collins C, Wang Y. High prevalence of tobacco use and exposure to secondhand tobacco smoke among adolescents in low- and middle-income countries. Ann Transl Med 2017;5(Suppl 1):S4.

[3] West R. Tobacco smoking: Health impact, prevalence, correlates and interventions. Psychol Health 2017;32(8):1018-36.

[4] Omaduvie U, Adisa A. Exposure to secondhand smoke in home and public areas among adolescents in Abuja, Nigeria: Tobacco control implications. Tobacco Prev Cessation 2015;1:8.

[5] Desalu OO, Onyedum CC, Adewole OO, Fawibe AE, Salami AK. Secondhand smoke exposure among nonsmoking adults in two Nigerian cities. Ann Afr Med 2011;10(2):103-11.

[6] Ekanem IA. Global youth tobacco survey for Nigeria report. Calabar, Cross-River State: Department of Pathology, 2008.

[7] Fagbule OF, Kanmodi KK, Aladelusi TO. Secondhand tobacco smoke exposure and attitudes towards tobacco ban: A pilot survey of secondary school students in Ibokun Town, Nigeria. Int J Child Adolesc Health 2018;11(3):349-53.

[8] Kanmodi KK, Fagbule OF, Aladelusi TO. Prevalence of shisha (waterpipe) smoking and awareness of head and neck cancer among Nigerian secondary school students: A preliminary survey. Int Public Health J 2018;10(2):210-4.

[9] Mohammed FA, Kanmodi KK, Fagbule OF, Adesina MA, Njideka NJ, Sadiq HA. Shisha smokers' desire to quit shisha smoking habit: findings from a Nigerian pilot survey. Global Psychiatry 2019;2(1):37-41.

[10] Aanyu C, Ddamulira JB, Nyamurungi K, Ediau M, Bazeyo W. Knowledge, attitudes and practices of Shisha smoking among youths in Kampala, Uganda. Tob Induc Dis 2018;16(Suppl 1):A484.

[11] Al-Naggar RA, Bobryshev YV, Anil S. Pattern of shisha and cigarette smoking in the general population in Malaysia. Asian Pac J Cancer Prev 2014;15(24):10841-6.

[12] Martinasek MP, McDermott RJ, Martini L. Waterpipe (hookah) tobacco smoking among youth. Curr Probl Pediatr Adolesc Health Care 2011;41:34-57.

[13] Mugyenyi AE, Haberer JE, O'Neil I. Pleasure and practice: a qualitative study of the individual and social underpinnings of shisha use in cafes among youth in the UK. BMJ Open 2018;8(4):e018989.

[14] Kadhum M, Sweidan A, Jaffery AE, Al-Saadi A, Madden B. A review of health effects of smoking shisha. Clin Med (Lond) 2015;15(3):263-6.

[15] Olowookere SA. Adepoju EG, Gbolahan OO. Awareness and attitude to the law banning smoking in public places in Osun State, Nigeria. Tob Induc Dis 2014;12(1):6.

[16] Kanmodi KK, Nnebedum N, Bello M, Adesina M, Fagbule OF, Adesoye O. Head and neck cancer awareness: A survey of young people in international communities. Int J Adolesc Med Health [Accepted].

[17] Adesina MA, Kanmodi KK, Fagbule OF, Ogunmuko T. Unfavorable family background is associated with smoking at youthful age. Int J Child Health Hum Dev 2019;12(2):In press.

[18] Maziak W, Eissenberg T, Ward KD. Patterns of waterpipe use and dependence: implications for intervention development. Pharmacol Biochem Behav 2005;80:173-9.

[19] Martinasek MP, McDermott RJ, Martini L. Waterpipe (hookah) tobacco smoking among youth. Curr Probl Pediatr Adolesc Health Care 2011;41:34-57.

[20] Afifi R, Khalil J, Fouad F, Hammal F, Jarallah Y, Abu Farhat H, et al. Social norms and attitudes linked to waterpipe use in the Eastern Mediterranean Region. Soc Sci Med 2013;98:125-34.

[21] Al-Naggar RA, Saghir FS. Water pipe (shisha) smoking and associated factors among Malaysian university students. Asian Pac J Cancer Prev 2011;12(11):3041-7.

[22] WHO Study Group on Tobacco Product Regulation (TobReg). Advisory note: Waterpipe tobacco smoking: health effects, research needs and recommended actions by regulators, 2nd ed. Geneva: World Health Organization; 2015.

[23] Mohammed FA, Njideka NJ, Aliyu BM, Kanmodi KK, Fagbule OF, Ogbeide ME. Attitudes of a snowballed sample of Nigerian hookah (shisha) smokers toward tobacco ban: A short report. Int J Disabil Hum Dev 2019;18(2):In press.

In: Nigeria: Perspectives of Health
Editors: Ariel Tenenbaum et al.
ISBN: 978-1-53618-090-9

Chapter 12

THE KNOWLEDGE OF DRUG PRESCRIBERS, DISPENSERS, AND ADMINISTERS IN SOKOTO METROPOLIS, NIGERIA, ON NON-OPIOID ANALGESICS: ANY NEED FOR A REFRESHER COURSE?

Kehinde K Kanmodi[1,2,3,*], BDS, Catherine Fidelis[4], BPharm and Johnson Olajolumo[5], MB, BS

[1]Cephas Health Research Initiative Inc, Sokoto
[2]Department of Dental and Maxillofacial Surgery, Usmanu Danfodiyo University Teaching Hospital, Sokoto, Nigeria
[3]Community Health Officers Training Programme, Usmanu Danfodiyo University Teaching Hospital, Sokoto, Nigeria
[4]Department of Pharmacy, Usmanu Danfodiyo University Teaching Hospital, Sokoto, Nigeria
[5]Department of Medicine, Obafemi Awolowo University Teaching Hospital, Ile-Ife, Nigeria

[*] Corresponding Author's Email: kanmodikehinde@yahoo.com.

Abstract

Pain management is a very important aspect in the holistic care of patients. The clinical practitioner's knowledge of the pharmacology of pain killers goes a long way in the effective control of pain. Objectives: To assess the level of knowledge of clinical practitioners in Sokoto metropolis, Nigeria, on the pharmacology of non-opioid analgesics (NOAs). Methods: This study utilized the primary data obtained from a cross-section of 175 clinical practitioners working in five randomly selected hospitals situated within the metropolitan city of Sokoto, Nigeria. The study tool was a 17-item questionnaire. Data analysis was done using the SPSS version 16 Software. Results: Less than four-tenth (36.5%) of the subjects were within the age bracket of 26 to 30 years. 62.3% were males, 45% were nursing officers, and 36% had less than six years of experience in clinical practice. None of the surveyed pharmacists strongly disagreed that they were knowledgeable about the metabolism of NOAs, unlike the subjects in other occupational categories ($p < 0.0001$, df = 12). All of the surveyed dentists knew of the World Health Organization (WHO) analgesic ladder, unlike the other subjects in the other occupational categories ($p = 0.001$, df = 12). A range of 30 to 40% of the nurses, medical doctors, and pharmacists surveyed in this study considered tramadol to be a NOA. Paracetamol, ibuprofen, and diclofenac were the top three commonly prescribed NOAs among the subjects. The most common side effects of NOAs known to the subjects were nausea, vomiting, and peptic ulcer disease (PUD). Conclusion: Many of the surveyed subjects had inadequate knowledge of NOAs. This study population will highly benefit from educational programs that are focused on the clinical use of NOAs.

Introduction

The knowledge of a clinical practitioner on the pharmacology of pain killers is very important in patient management. In fact, it is virtually impossible for a practicing clinical practitioner not to prescribe, administer or dispense analgesic medications in his/her entire lifetime of clinical practice; hence this reflects the need for a clinical practitioner to have a very sound knowledge on pain management.

Pain can be managed pharmacologically and/or non-pharmacologically (1-5). The pharmacological management of pain involves the use of drugs

(1, 2), while the non-pharmacological management involves the use of other means, such as acupuncture, acupressure, behavioral therapy, and physical therapy (3-5).

One of the main groups of drugs used in the pharmacological management of pain is known as analgesics (1, 2). The analgesics are broadly classified into the opioid analgesics (OAs) and the non-opioid analgesics (NOAs). The OAs are known to be more potent in pain control than the NOAs (6); however one of the major problems associated with the use of OAs is the risk of dependence or tolerance (7).

It is an unbeatable fact that the NOAs still remain as the most commonly prescribed analgesics globally. After thorough literature search, authors noticed that the majority of the available literatures assessing clinicians' knowledge of analgesics were focused on OAs while only few literatures assessed clinicians' knowledge of NOAs. This study aims to assess the level of knowledge of doctors, nurses, and pharmacists in Sokoto metropolis, Nigeria, on the pharmacology of NOAs. Conducting this kind of study among this population group is of high significance as the outcome of the study will provide information on how knowledgeable they are on the pharmacology of NOAs.

OUR STUDY

This was a cross-sectional study conducted under the ethical guidelines of the Helsinki Declaration on health research involving human subjects. Approval to conduct this study was officially obtained from the Ethical Clearance Committee, Ministry of Health, Sokoto State, Nigeria (Ref. No: SKHREC/068/017). All subject participation was absolutely voluntary, and all identities were kept strictly confidential.

The instrument used for data collection was an anonymous well-structured 17-item questionnaire. This questionnaire had three sections. The first section obtained information on the bio-data of the participants. The second section obtained information from the participants on their knowledge of the: pharmacology (route of administration, dosage, and, adverse effects) of NOAs; and management of complications associated with NOA overdose. The third section obtained information from the participants on the frequency at which they prescribe NOAs to patients.

This study was a survey of nurses, medical doctors, pharmacists, and dentists working in five hospitals situated within the metropolitan city of Sokoto, Nigeria. A total of 188 consenting participants were recruited for this study using simple random sampling technique. Each of the participants was issued a paper questionnaire to fill and return. Only 175 (93.1%) out of the 188 participants returned their questionnaires filled. None of the returned questionnaires was discarded, because all were properly filled.

Data analysis was done using the SPSS version 20 software. The frequency distributions of all variables were determined, and tests of associations between variables were done using the Chi-square test with a p-value of < 0.05 considered to be of statistical significance. The statistical results obtained were presented using tables.

FINDINGS

About four-tenth (36.5%) of the 175 subjects were within the age bracket of 26 to 30 years. 62.3% were males, 45% were nursing officers, and 36% of them had less than six years of experience in clinical practice (see Table 1). None of the surveyed pharmacists strongly disagreed that they were knowledgeable about the metabolism of NOAs, unlike the subjects in other occupational categories ($p < 0.0001$, df = 12). Furthermore, less than 40% of all the subjects in each occupational category strongly agreed that they knew the dosage of NOAs ($p = 0.066$, df = 12). It is also noteworthy that all of the surveyed dentists knew of the World Health Organization (WHO) analgesic ladder, unlike other subjects in the other occupational categories ($p = 0.001$, df = 12) (see Table 2). Interestingly, a range of 30 to 40% of the nurses, medical doctors, and pharmacists surveyed in this study considered tramadol to be a NOA (see Table 3).

Table 1. Bio-data of the subjects (n = 175)

Characteristics	**Frequency (%)**
Gender	
Male	109 (62.3)
Female	66 (37.7)
Age (in years)	
< 21	1 (0.6)
21 – 25	20 (11.4)
26 – 30	64 (36.5)
31 – 35	51 (29.1)
36 – 40	25 (14.3)
41 – 45	7 (4.0)
>46	6 (3.4)
Not specified	1 (0.6)
Year(s) of practice	
< 1	45 (25.7)
1 – 5	63 (36.0)
6 – 10	47 (26.9)
11 – 15	11 (6.3)
16 – 20	3 (1.7)
>20	5 (2.9)
Not specified	1 (0.6)
Profession	
Nurse	78 (45.0)
Medical doctor	62 (35.0)
Dentist	7 (4)
Pharmacist	28 (16)

Amidst other findings presented in Table 4, it is noteworthy that just only 9.0% and 7.1% of the surveyed nurses and pharmacists, respectively, did not prescribe NOAs to patients (see Table 4).

Paracetamol, ibuprofen, and diclofenac were the top three commonly prescribed NOAs among the subjects (see Table 5). The three most common side effects of NOAs known to the subjects were nausea, vomiting, and peptic ulcer disease (PUD) (see Table 6).

Lastly, the three most common route of administration of NOAs known by the subjects were intramuscular, intravenous, and the oral routes (see Table 7).

Table 2. Knowledge of the subjects about the pharmacology of NOAs and the clinical management of NOA overdose

Questions	Profession of respondents					
	Response	Nurse (N = 78)*	Medical doctor (N = 62)*	Dentist (N = 7)*	Pharmacist (N = 28)*	X2
I am knowledgeable about the metabolism of NOAs	SD	5 (6.4)	3 (4.8)	1 (14.3)	0 (0.0)	< 0.0001, df = 12
	D	11 (14.1)	3(4.8)	0(0.0)	0(0.0)	
	U	21 (26.9)	5(7.7)	0(0.0)	2(7.1)	
	A	40 (51.3)	33 (53.2)	5 (71.4)	17 (60.7)	
	SA	1 (1.3)	18 (29.0)	1 (14.3)	9 (32.1)	
	Total	78 (100.0)	62(100.0)	7(100.0)	28(100.0)	
I am knowledgeable about the dosage of NOAs	SD	6(7.7)	3(4.8)	1(14.3)	1(3.6)	0.066, df = 12
	D	5(6.4)	0(0.0)	0(0.0)	0(0.0)	
	U	11(14.1)	2(3.2)	0(0.0)	1(3.6)	
	A	42(53.8)	36(58.1)	3(0.0)	15(53.6)	
	SA	14(17.9)	21(33.9)	3(0.0)	11(39.3)	
	Total	78(100.0)	62(100.0)	7(100.0)	28(100.0)	
I am knowledgeable about the WHO analgesic ladder	Yes	34(43.6)	46(74.2)	7(100.0)	22(78.6)	0.001, df = 12
	No	27(34.6)	12(19.4)	0(0.0)	3(10.7)	
	Not sure	17(21.8)	4(6.5)	0(0.0)	3(10.7)	
	Total	78(100.0)	62(100.0)	7(100.0)	28(100.0)	
I know how to manage the complications of NOA overdose	SD	5(6.4)	2()	0(0.0)	0(0.0)	0.251, df = 12
	D	7(9.0)	1(1.6)	0(0.0)	0(0.0)	
	U	14(17.9)	10(16.1)	0(0.0)	5(0.0)	
	A	45(57.7)	36(58.1)	5(71.4)	19(23.2)	
	SA	7(9.0)	13(21.0)	2(28.6)	4(14.3)	
	Total	78(100.0)	62(100.0)	7(100.0)	28(100.0)	

N = Total number of respondents in each category; SD = Strongly disagree; D = Disagree; U = Undecided; A = agree; SA = Strongly agree; X^2 = Chi square; df = Degree of freedom.

Table 3. Knowledge of the subjects on the drug class of tramadol

Question		Profession of respondents					
		Nurse (N = 78)	Medical doctor (N = 62)	Dentist (N = 7)	Pharmacist (N = 28)	Total (N = 175)	X2
Tramadol is a NOA	Yes	30 (38.5)	19 (30.6)	0 (0.0)	4 (14.3)	53 (30.3)	< 0.0001, df = 6
	No	27 (34.5)	40 (64.5)	7 (100.0)	22 (78.6)	96 (54.9)	
	Not sure	21 (26.9)	3 (4.8)	0 (0.0)	2 (7.1)	26 (14.9)	
	Total	78 (100.0)	62 (100.0)	7 (100.0)	28 (100.0)	175 (100.0)	

N = Total number of respondents in each category; X2 = Chi square; df = Degree of freedom.

Table 4. Comparison between the frequency of NOA prescription and the profession of the subjects

Question		Profession of respondents					
		Nurse (N = 78)	Medical doctor	Dentist	Pharmacist	Total	X2
How often do you prescribe NOA to patients?	Never	7(9.0)	0(0.0)	0(0.0)	2(7.1)	9(5.1)	0.018, df = 12
	Rare	12(15.4)	1(1.6)	0(0.0)	5(17.9)	18(10.3)	
	Sometimes	33(42.3)	25(40.3)	2(28.6)	9(32.1)	69(39.4)	
	Usually	17(21.8)	25(40.3)	2(28.6)	9(32.1)	53(30.3)	
	Always	9(11.5)	11(17.7)	3(42.9)	3(10.7)	26(14.9)	
	Total	78(100.0)	62(100.0)	7(100.0)	28(100.0)	175(100.0)	

Table 5. Response of the subjects to the question: Can you mention three NOA you commonly prescribe to patients?

Drugs indicated	Profession of respondents				
	Nurse	Medical doctor	Dentist	Pharmacist	Total
Dihydrocodeine	1	1	0	0	2
Morphine	2	0	0	0	2
Paraldehyde	1	0	0	0	1
Tramadol	11	7	0	0	18
Tenoxicam	0	1	0	2	3
Diclofenac	36	44	7	22	109
Mefenamic acid	0	2	0	0	2
Hyoscine hydrobromide	0	2	0	0	2
Pentazocine	4	1	0	0	5
Indomethacin	2	1	0	0	3
Ibuprofen	46	35	5	23	109
Dipyrone	1	0	0	0	1
Piroxicam	18	17	0	6	41
Paracetamol	52	37	5	17	111
Aceclofenac	0	4	1	4	9
Naproxen	0	4	0	1	5
Meloxicam	0	3	1	0	4
Celecoxib	2	2	0	1	5
Ketorolac	0	2	0	0	2
Aspirin	17	10	2	2	31

Table 6. Response of the subjects to the question: Can you list six (6) adverse effects of NOAs?

Side effects	Profession of respondents				
	Nurse	Medical doctors	Dentist	Pharmacist	Total
General					
Fatigue	3	0	0	0	3
Hypothermia	2	0	0	0	2
Malaise	0	0	0	1	1
Weakness	11	0	0	0	11
Edema	0	0	0	2	2
Restlessness	1	0	0	0	1
Hyperactivity	1	0	0	0	1
Cardiovascular					
Cardiac toxicity	0	1	0	0	1
Hypertension	2	6	0	4	12
Heart failure	1	0	0	0	1
Premature closure of PDA	0	4	0	1	5
Abnormal heart rate	0	0	0	1	1

Side effects	Profession of respondents				
	Nurse	Medical doctors	Dentist	Pharmacist	Total
Gastrointestinal					
Indigestion	1	0	0	0	1
Heart burn	7	2	1	1	11
Nausea	35	27	4	13	79
Hepatotoxicity	2	10	2	5	19
Hepatitis	0	0	1	3	4
Liver failure	0	5	0	0	5
Liver cancer	0	0	1	0	1
GERD	0	0	0	1	1
Anorexia	4	0	1	1	6
Vomiting	36	20	3	10	69
Abdominal discomfort	14	7	0	9	30
Abdominal pain	5	4	1	2	12
Dyspepsia	3	2	1	1	7
Melena	0	1	0	0	1
Oesophagitis	0	1	0	0	1
Esophageal ulcer	0	1	0	0	1
Constipation	15	6	0	2	23
Diarrhea	10	3	1	4	18
Gastritis	0	13	0	0	13
Gastric cancer	0	1	0	0	1
Hyperacidity	4	0	0	0	4
PUD	6	32	4	15	57
Xerostomia	6	1	0	0	7
Urogenital					
Chronic kidney disease	0	1	0	0	1
Fluid retention	0	0	1	0	1
Urinary intention	1	1	0	1	3
Renal tubular necrosis	0	1	0	0	1
Nephropathy	0	4	0	0	4
Nephrotoxicity	1	11	3	5	20
Acute kidney injury	0	4	0	0	4
Hematological					
Acidosis	1	0	0	0	1
Blood intoxication	1	0	0	0	1
Hemorrhage	9	25	3	12	49
Coagulopathy	0	2	0	0	2
Pancytopenia	0	1	0	0	1
Platelet dysfunction	0	6	0	0	6
Neutropenia	0	1	0	0	1
Blood dyscrasia	1	0	0	0	1
Neurological					
Confusion	2	0	0	1	3
Headache	9	5	1	5	20
Raised ICP	1	0	0	0	1

Table 6. (Continued)

Side effects	Profession of respondents				
	Nurse	Medical doctors	Dentist	Pharmacist	Total
Insomnia	2	0	0	0	2
Light-headedness	0	0	0	2	2
Loss of consciousness	2	0	0	0	2
Reye syndrome	0	3	0	1	4
Irritability	1	0	0	0	1
Drowsiness	16	3	0	0	19
Vertigo	0	0	0	1	1
Dizziness	18	8	1	9	36
Convulsion	1	1	0	0	2
Nervous disorder	0	1	0	0	1
Cognitive impairment	4	1	0	0	5
Sedation	1	0	0	0	1
Ophthalmologic					
Blurred vision	2	0	0	0	2
Behavioral					
Hallucination	2	0	0	0	2
Euphoria	1	0	0	0	1
Addiction	4	9	1	0	14
Tolerance	1	1	0	0	2
Irrational talk	2	0	0	0	2
Anxiety	2	0	0	2	4
Dermatological					
Angioedema	0	1	0	0	1
Pruritus	6	1	1	0	8
Urticaria	0	6	1	3	10
Itching	4	0	1	0	5
Otorhinolaryngological					
Tinnitus	1	1	1	0	3
Immunological					
Steven-Johnson syndrome	0	3	1	3	7
Allergy	1	5	2	1	9
Hypersensitivity reaction	1	2	0	1	4
Anaphylactic reaction	1	1	0	0	2
Respiratory					
Asthma	0	8	0	4	12
Respiratory depression	3	1	0	0	4
Others					
Tissue necrosis	1	0	0	0	1
Drug interaction	0	1	0	0	1
Metabolic disorders	1	0	0	0	1

PDA = Patent ductus arteriosus; GERD = Gastroesophageal reflux disease; ICP = Intracranial pressure; PUD = Peptic ulcer disease.

Table 7. Response of the subjects to the question: Can you list seven (7) routes of administration of NOAs?

Routes of administration indicated by respondents	Profession of respondents				
	Nurse	Medical doctor	Dentist	Pharmacist	Total
Intravenous	65	53	7	26	151
Intramuscular	61	55	7	27	150
Intra-articular	0	2	1	0	3
Intra-mucosal	2	1	0	0	3
Buccal	0	0	1	0	1
Oral	71	55	7	27	160
Intra-capsular	0	1	0	0	1
Superficial	3	0	0	0	3
Drop	0	1	0	0	1
Sublingual	7	15	2	2	26
Intra-vaginal	3	0	0	0	3
Intra-peritoneal	0	1	0	0	1
Rectal	38	30	3	20	91
Topical	21	26	1	9	57
Intra-thecal	9	9	0	2	20
Intra-nasal	1	3	0	0	4
Otic route	1	0	0	0	1
Transdermal	16	10	4	9	39
Intra-cordal	1	0	0	1	2
Subcutaneous	17	8	3	5	33
Inhalational	8	1	0	1	10
Epidural	0	1	0	1	2
Intra-osseus	0	0	1	0	1
Spray	5	2	0	0	7
Aerosol	2	0	0	0	2
Intra-lesional	0	1	0	0	1
Intra-ocular	1	2	5	0	8

DISCUSSION

This study surveyed a sample of nurses, dentists, medical doctors, and pharmacists working in five major hospitals situated within the metropolitan city of Sokoto, Nigeria, on their knowledge of the pharmacology of NOAs. The significance of this study was that it provided information on subjects' level of knowledge on NOAs (the NOAs are the first line of drugs in pain management (8)).

Pain is a common symptom in many disease conditions. In patient management, pain control is a very important aspect that needs to be put into consideration. Pain management in a hospital setting involves a multidisciplinary approach. Starting from the doctor, after clinical diagnosis has been made, analgesics are prescribed to the patient in a prescription note. Thereafter, the drugs are dispensed by the pharmacist before being finally administered by the nurse.

Based on the above, a clinical practitioner needs to have a very sound knowledge of the pharmacology of NOAs. From the findings made in this study, it can be said that the knowledge of many of the subjects was inadequate. First of all, not all of them had sound knowledge of the metabolism and dosage of NOAs. This is noteworthy because these individuals are actively involved in patient management; hence their knowledge deficits in pain management may tell negatively on the proper management of their patient.

Secondly, some of the subjects did not know the class of analgesics where tramadol belongs to, as many of them considered tramadol to be a NOA. Tramadol is an OA which is known to cause dependence (9, 10); it is also one of the abused drugs in the environment where this study was carried out (11). Unfortunately, the wrong understanding of tramadol as a NOA among the subjects might have made some of them prescribed this drug irrationally to patients increasing such patients' level of risk of developing drug addiction to tramadol.

Thirdly, some of the subjects demonstrated poor knowledge of the adverse effects of NOAs. For instance, some of them mentioned addiction, tolerance, euphoria, and hallucination as adverse effects of NOA, meanwhile NOAs are not known to have addictive or psychedelic effect (12, 13). Furthermore, the most commonly prescribed drugs among the respondents were ibuprofen, diclofenac, and paracetamol. Diclofenac and Ibuprofen are popularly known to cause drug-induced peptic ulcer (14); possibly, some of these respondents may not know of this adverse effect.

Fourthly, some of the subjects in this present study had poor knowledge about the route of administration of NOAs. It is noteworthy that some of them highlighted some wrong routes of administration such as "spray," "epidural," "intra-vaginal," and "intra-capsular," to mention a few.

Based on the above findings, authors conclude that the surveyed clinical practitioners in this present study demonstrated inadequate knowledge of the pharmacology of NOAs. Authors would like to recommend that continual medical education (CME) programs (such as workshops, and seminars) on the use of NOAs should be organized for this population group. By doing so, their knowledge will be updated on the use of these drugs in patient management; hence improving the quality of services they render to the sick.

ACKNOWLEDGMENTS

Authors declare that they have no competing interest regarding this study.

REFERENCES

[1] Park HJ, Moon DE. Pharmacologic management of chronic pain. Korean J Pain 2010; 23(2):99-108.

[2] Ahmadi A, Bazargan-Hejazi S, Heidari Zadie Z, Euasohon P, Ketumarn P, et al. Pain management in trauma: A review study. J Inj Violence Res 2016;8(2):89-98.

[3] Amatya B, Young J, Khan F. Non-pharmacological interventions for chronic pain in multiple sclerosis (Protocol). Cochrane Database Syst Rev 2017;3:CD012622.

[4] Chang KL, Fillingim R, Hurley RW, Schmidt S. Chronic pain management: nonpharmacological therapies for chronic pain. FP Essent 2015;432:21-6.

[5] Pak SC, Micalos PS, Maria SJ, Lord B. Nonpharmacological interventions for pain management in paramedicine and the emergency setting: a review of the literature. Evid Based Complementary Altern Med 2015;2015:873039.

[6] Schung SA, Garrett WB, Gillespie G. Opioid and non-opioid analgesics. Best Pract Res Clin Anaesthiol 2003;17(1):91-110.

[7] Labianca R, Sarzi-Puttini P, Zuccaro SM, Cherubino P, Vellucci R, Fornasari D. Adverse effects associated with non-opioid treatment in patients with chronic pain. Clin Drug Investig 2012;32(Suppl 1):53-63.

[8] World Health Organization. WHO's cancer pain ladder for adults, 2017. URL: www.who.int/cancer/palliative/painladder/en/

[9] Minami K, Uezono Y, Ueta Y. Pharmacological aspects of the effects of tramadol on G-protein coupled receptors. J Pharmacol Sci 2007;103(3):253-60.

[10] Zabihi E, Hoseinzaadeh A, Emami M, Mardani M, Mahmoud B, Akbar MA. Potential for tramadol abuse by patients visiting pharmacies in northern Iran. Subst Abuse 2011;5:11-5.

[11] Ibrahim AW, Yerima MM, Pindar SK, Onyencho VC, Ahmed HK, et al. Tramadol abuse among patients attending an addiction clinic in North-Eastern Nigeria: outcome of a four year retrospective study. Adv Psychol Neurosci 2017;2(2):31-37.

[12] Cashman JN. The mechanisms of action of NSAIDs in analgesia. Drugs 1996;52(Suppl 5):13-23.

[13] Graham GG, Scott KE. Mechanism of action of paracetamol. Am J Ther 2005;12(1):46-55.

[14] Drini M. Peptic ulcer disease and non-steroidal anti-inflammatory drugs. Aust Prescr 2017;40(3):91-3.

In: Nigeria: Perspectives of Health
Editors: Ariel Tenenbaum et al.
ISBN: 978-1-53618-090-9

Chapter 13

NECK CIRCUMFERENCE AS A SCREENING INSTRUMENT FOR OVERWEIGHT AND OBESITY IN NIGERIAN SECONDARY SCHOOL ADOLESCENTS IN AN URBAN AREA

Eden E Igbafe[1,*], MBBS, MPH, FMCPaed, Mike N Ibeabuchi[2], MBBS, MSc, PhD, MPA, Elizabeth E Oyenusi[3,4], MBBS, FMCPaed, MWACP, FESPE, Abiola Oduwole[3,4], MBBS, FWACP and James Renner[5], MBBS, FMCPaed

[1]Department of Paediatrics, Nigerian Air Force Hospital, Ikeja, Lagos, [2]Department of Anatomy, College of Medicine, University of Lagos, Lagos, [3]Department of Paediatrics, College of Medicine, University of Lagos, Lagos, [4]Paediatric Endocrinology Training Centre for West Africa, Lagos University Teaching Hospital, Idi-araba, Lagos and [5] Department of Paediatrics, Babcock University, Ilishan, Ogun State, Nigeria

---

[*] Corresponding Author's Email: eden_igbafe@yahoo.com.

ABSTRACT

Overweight and obesity are on the increase worldwide and the adolescent population is of special concern. Methods of assessing overweight and obesity are being explored but neck circumference has not been widely investigated in adolescents. Objective: This study aimed at assessing neck circumference as a simple screening tool for overweight and obesity among Nigerian adolescents. Study group and Methods: A cross sectional survey was conducted among 897 adolescents aged 10-19 years in urban Lagos, using a stratified, multistage sampling method. Overweight and obesity were defined using the criteria by the United States Center for Disease Control. Student t test was used for continuous data and Pearson correlation coefficient for exploring the relationship between neck circumference and other variables. Receiver operating characteristic analysis was used to evaluate optimal neck circumference cutoffs for overweight or obesity. Results: 64 adolescents (7.1%) were overweight while those with obesity were 33 (3.7%). Neck circumference was positively correlated with age and Body Mass Index. There were significant differences in the neck circumferences of those that were overweight or with obesity compared to those with normal weight. The cutoff ranges for overweight/obesity per adolescent period were 33.95 to 36.95cm in males and 31.05 to 33.40cm in females. Sensitivities were 70-96.6% while specificities were 60.2-87.7%. Conclusions: Neck circumference is a simple and reliable tool which could be used to screen for overweight and obesity in Nigerian adolescents.

INTRODUCTION

Overweight and obesity have become major public concerns worldwide (1) as they are being reported increasingly in developed and recently in developing countries (2) including Nigeria (3). The adolescent population is of special concern because the health and mortality risks of these phenomena are higher when developed during this period compared to development in adulthood (4). Therefore, screening and detection of adolescent overweight and obesity are important as there are strategies to manage them (4). Furthermore, a preliminary step towards curtailing the obesity epidemic is to provide monitoring tools that are cost effective, quick, easy to use, and acceptable to both recipients and health care practitioners (1).

Weight status is currently being described using the body mass index (BMI) (5), which in children and adolescents, varies with age and gender (5). It has however been criticized for its reduced ability to describe central fat with which the greater health risks of overweight and obesity are associated (6) and for its time consuming derivation (7), amongst other things. Hence, simple, acceptable, quick and reliable methods of assessing overweight and obesity are being explored (7).

The neck is an easily accessible part of the body and its measurement is simple, quick and inexpensive (1, 7). Limited studies have been documented on the use of neck circumference (NC), to identify overweight and obesity (1, 7, 8). However, NC has not been investigated as a screening tool for overweight and obesity in Nigerian adolescents. The aim of this study is to determine the usefulness of neck circumference as a screening tool for overweight and obesity among Nigerian adolescents.

OUR SURVEY

A cross sectional survey was conducted from March to July 2013, among a representative sample of 897 adolescents aged 10-19 years in urban Lagos, using a stratified, multistage sampling method. Metropolitan Lagos is said to have captured 36.8% of Nigeria's urban population (9) making it the nation's largest urban population. The multistage sampling method included simple random, stratified random, systematic random and probability proportional-to-size (PPS) sampling techniques employed in the different stages.

Ethical and administrative approvals were obtained from the Health Research and Ethics Committee of the Lagos University Teaching Hospital and the Lagos State Ministry of Education, respectively.

Only those who satisfied the inclusion criteria were enrolled for the study. These criteria included subjects in the age group 10-19 years, consent from parents or guardians, assent from subjects and completed questionnaires. Exclusion criteria applied were possession of neck masses or deformities and history of or features suggestive of chronic ill health such as sickle cell disease and poorly controlled bronchial asthma.

Measurements

The selected study participants had their anthropometries determined. Trained volunteer measurers took the anthropometric measurements which included weight, height and neck circumference. These three measurements were taken using standard methods, according to the protocols recommended in the International Standards for Anthropometric Assessment published (10).

Body Mass Index (BMI)

BMI was calculated using a standard formula:

BMI = Weight (kg)/height^2 (m^2) in kg/m^2

This was done with the aid of the Children's BMI Tool for Schools (11), a software produced by the United States Centre for Disease Control. Adolescents with BMI at 85th to just below the 95th percentile were said to be with overweight while those with BMI at 95th percentile and above were with obesity.

Data analysis

The data was analyzed using the statistical software package SSPS Version 17.0. Mean with standard deviation were generated as necessary for age and gender specific anthropometric indices. Tests of statistical significance included Student's t test for continuous data and chi-square test for discrete data. Pearson correlation coefficient was used to explore the association between neck circumference and other continuous variables.

Receiver operating characteristic (ROC) analyses were used to determine the predictive validity of neck circumference and also evaluate optimal cut off values for adolescents with overweight and obesity in the different age categories. ROC curves assess the ability of a screening test to diagnose an outcome correctly, with reference to a gold standard.

The essentials of ROC analysis include (12) the sensitivity, specificity, the positive (PPV) or negative predictive value (NPV) of the test, the likelihood ratio for a positive (LR+) or a negative (LR-) test, the ROC curve and its area under the curve (AUC). Sensitivity and specificity are usefully combined in likelihood ratios. A high likelihood ratio for a positive result and a low likelihood ratio for a negative result indicate that a test is useful (12). The ideal test would have an AUC of 1 while a random guess would have an AUC of 0.5. Hence, AUC values closer to 1 indicate a test is useful. Probability values less than 0.05 were accepted as statistically significant.

FINDINGS

Eight hundred and ninety-seven students, selected from public and private schools, participated in the study. Of these, ninety seven were either overweight or obese based on defined BMI criteria (11), making the overall prevalence of overweight and obesity 10.8%. Prevalence of obesity was 3.7% (thirty-three) while that of overweight was 7.1% (sixty-four).

Body mass index categories in relation to gender (see table 1)

This shows the overall prevalence of overweight and obesity along gender lines.

Table 1. Body mass index categories in relation to gender

	BMI Percentile		
Gender	**<85th Percentile**	**≥85th Percentile**	**Total**
Female	474 (87.13%)	70 (12.87%)	544 (100%)
Male	326 (92.35%)	27 (7.65%)	353 (100%)
Total	800 (89.2%)	97 (10.8%)	897 (100%)

Chi-square test ($\times^2$): 6.046, p value = 0.014.

Table 2. The neck circumference of study participants in relation to age and gender

		Male		Female		
Age (years)	**n**	**Mean (± SD) cm**	**n**	**Mean (± SD)cm**	**t**	**p**
10	12	30.49 (2.50)	12	30.50 (1.76)	-0.021	0.98
11	23	29.68 (2.86)	39	30.15 (2.81)	0.436	0.67
12	48	30.80 (2.34)	83	30.80 (2.58)	-1.014	0.316
13	48	31.68 (2.87)	88	30.86 (2.18)	-1.046	0.301
14	44	32.19 (2.78)	84	30.48 (2.09)	-3.306	0.002
15	60	33.30 (2.80)	109	31.34 (2.33)	-4.042	<0.001
16	51	34.11 (2.58)	66	31.17 (2.23)	-6.454	<0.001
17	37	35.09 (2.55)	34	31.37 (2.14)	-7.496	<0.001
18	20	34.87 (2.04)	20	31.32 (2.22)	-6.697	<0.001
19	10	36.85 (3.83)	9	31.94 (3.27)	-2.708	0.027
All	353	32.77 (3.17)	544	30.93 (2.35)		

Neck circumference range in relation to age and gender (see table 2)

The mean NC (± S.D) for all males 32.77(3.17) cm while that for all females was 30.93(2.35) cm. From the ages of 10 to 13 years, the mean NC values in males and females were not significantly different. However, from the age of 14 to 19 years, the mean NC values of males were significantly higher than those of females ($p < 0.001$ to $p = 0.027$).

Neck circumference range in relation to age, gender and body mass index categories (see table 3)

Table 3 shows that the mean NC (± S.D) of all adolescent males with BMI <85th percentile was 30.05(2.03) cm while in those with BMI ≥85th percentile it was 35.5(3.09) cm (p = <0.001). For the adolescent females, these were 29.23(1.95) cm and 33.76(2.54) cm respectively (p = <0.001). Thus, there was a significant difference in the NC of subjects in the two BMI categories in both genders.

Table 3. Neck circumference of study participants in relation to age, gender and body mass index categories

Age (years)	Males				Females			
	<85th percentile		**≥85th percentile**		**<85th percentile**		**≥85th percentile**	
	Mean (± SD)cm	**n**	**Mean (±SD)cm**	**n**	**Mean (± SD)cm**	**n**	**Mean (± SD)cm**	**n**
10	30.10 (1.49)	10	32.55 (2.05)	2	29.26 (1.72)	8	32.95 (1.98)	4
11	29.50 (2.92)	21	31.60 (0.42)	2	29.28 (2.06)	31	33.61 (2.59)	8
12	30.56 (2.13)	45	34.46 (2.75)	3	30.18 (1.83)	72	34.84 (3.07)	11
13	31.34 (2.63)	42	34.10 (3.58)	6	30.73 (2.19)	82	32.72 (1.45)	6
14	31.94 (2.56)	42	37.45 (2.19)	2	30.13 (1.79)	75	33.23 (2.46)	9
15	33.02 (2.69)	55	36.40 (2.31)	5	30.96 (1.99)	94	33.69 (2.88)	15
16	33.89 (2.39)	49	39.35 (1.06)	2	30.75 (1.81)	59	34.71 (2.45)	7
17	34.73 (2.46)	32	37.34 (1.98)	5	30.72 (1.48)	26	33.48 (2.68)	8
18	34.86 (2.04)	20	- -		31.04 (2.17)	18	33.75 (0.35)	2
19	36.85 (3.83)	10	- -		31.94 (3.27)	9	- -	
All	30.05 (2.03)	326	35.50 (3.09)	27	29.23 (1.95)	474	33.76 (2.54)	70

t test: -7.328, p < 0.001 (Males)
t test: -10.824, p < 0.001 (Females)

Correlation studies

There was significant positive correlation between neck circumference and BMI (r = 0.538, p < 0.001). When split along gender lines and adolescent periods the correlation is shown in Table 4.

Table 4. Correlation between neck circumference and body mass index in relation to gender and period of adolescence

Age group	Male r	p value	Female r	p value
10 – 13 years	0.556	<0.001	0.673	<0.001
14 – 16 years	0.698	<0.001	0.650	<0.001
17 – 19 years	0.515	<0.001	0.554	<0.001

Optimal cutoff values of neck circumference for overweight/obesity

Table 5 shows the AUC and NC cutoff values with their corresponding sensitivities and specificities in the males per adolescent period. Using the ROC statistical maneuvers, the optimal NC cutoff for overweight and obesity in a boy in middle adolescence is 35.85cm with a sensitivity of 77.8% and specificity of 87.7%. The positive likelihood ratio (LR+) of 6.3, indicates that a boy of 14-16 years with a NC greater than 35.85cm is 6.3 times more likely to be with overweight or obesity than a boy of the same age with NC value less than or equal to 35.85cm. A negative likelihood ratio (LR-) of 0.2 means that a negative result (≤ 35.85cm) is 0.2 times as likely for a 14-16 year old boy who is overweight or obese as one who is normal weight. Table 6 shows the AUC and NC cutoff values with their corresponding sensitivities and specificities in the females per adolescent period. As was done in the males, the optimal NC cutoff for overweight and obesity in a girl in early adolescence is 31.05cm with a sensitivity of 96.6% and specificity of 65.8%. Also, the LR+ of a girl of in this group (10-13 years) with a NC of > 31.05cm is 2.8 while LR- is 0.05. Furthermore, though the sensitivities of the proposed cutoff values decrease as age increases, their LR+ are almost the same or increase with a corresponding decrease in LR-, indicating their usefulness.

Table 5. Optimal neck circumference cutoff values for high body mass index in males, their sensitivities and specificities per adolescent period

Age group n(n^0) (years)	AUC (95% CI)	Cutoff (cm)	Sensitivity (%)	Specificity (%)	PPV (%)	NPV (%)	LR+	LR-
10 – 13 131(13)	0.786 (0.660-0.911)	31.05	84.6	60.2	19.1	97.4	2.1	0.49
14 – 16 155(9)	0.888 (0.786-0.990)	35.85	77.8	87.7	28.1	98.5	6.3	0.25
17 – 19 67(5)	0.774 (0.623-0.926)	36.05	80	69.4	16.7	97.8	2.6	0.29

n(n^0): total number (number with overweight/obesity), CI: Confidence Interval.

Table 6.Optimal neck circumference cutoff values for high body mass index in females, their sensitivities and specificities per adolescent period

Age group n(n^0) (years)	AUC (95% CI)	Cutoff (cm)	Sensitivity (%)	Specificity (%)	PPV (%)	NPV (%)	LR+	LR-
10 – 13 222(29)	0.877 (0.825-0.929)	31.05	96.6	65.8	29.8	99.2	2.8	0.05
14 – 16 259(31)	0.834 (0.760-0.908)	31.35	80.6	67.1	25.0	96.2	2.4	0.28
17 – 19 63(10)	0.802 (0.650-0.959)	32.90	70	84.9	46.9	93.7	4.6	0.35

n (n^0): total number (number of adolescents with overweight/obesity), CI: Confidence Interval.

DISCUSSION

There has been a rising trend in the prevalence of adolescent overweight and obesity globally (13). This poses major public health concerns because of the adverse associated outcomes such as psychosocial (14), health and socioeconomic consequences (15). Therefore, the importance of providing tools that screen and detect these epidemics cannot be over emphasized (1).

Various methods are available to assess body fat and thereby detect overweight or obesity, but for epidemiological purposes, body mass index(BMI) skin-fold thickness measurement, bioelectrical impedance analysis (BIA), waste circumference and waist–hip ratio are some which have been recommended (5, 16 17).

BMI, derived from weight and height, is currently the best available anthropometric estimate of fatness for public health purposes (18) and was used as the gold standard for overweight and obesity in this study. It has the advantages of being simple, easily available, inexpensive, with a high degree of reproducibility but limited because it does not discriminate between fat and muscle, does not correlate with central fat (the index of obesity related health risks) (18) and its derivation is time consuming (7).

BIA, a non-anthropometric tool, is relatively inexpensive (when compared with other non-anthropometric methods) and easy to use (16), but its results are influenced by the environment, ethnicity, phase of menstrual cycle and underlying medical conditions. Hence its measurements should be validated for specific ethnic groups, populations and conditions prior to its use (19).

Waist circumference (WC), an index of central fat distribution, also said to be the best simple anthropometric measure of total body fat and more sensitive than BMI (17) has limited wide-spread acceptance because there is no agreement about landmarks, when to measure it, and what it means (20). Furthermore, it could be culturally or environmentally problematic as clothes have to be removed for it to be measured accurately (1).

Neck circumference (NC), an index of central fat distribution, was found to be independently related to cardiovascular risk factors in obese adults (21), reported to be a simple and time-saving tool for screening and identifying overweight and obese adults (7) and children (1). Though said to correlate less with BMI than WC (1, 8), NC, unlike WC, has agreed land marks, is easily accessible in the neck, and clothes don't need to be removed for it to be measured accurately. Lastly, in adolescents, NC was found to show very good inter and intra-rater reliability (22). Multiple measurements are not required for precision and reliability.

In Nigeria, there's a dearth of studies on indices of central fat in the adolescent population and none has explored the usefulness of NC as a screening tool for overweight and obesity in adolescents, hence the relevance of this study.

This study confirms the presence of adolescent overweight and obesity in Nigeria, albeit at lower rates when compared with the western world and Mediterranean region, consistent with the review stating that countries in sub-Saharan Africa have the lowest prevalent rates of adolescent overweight and obesity (13). This is because the speed of this epidemic is said to be slower in less economically developed countries predominant in sub-Saharan Africa as a result of the less rapid changes in diet and activity associated with the lower income in these countries (13).

In this study, the mean NC of males and females aged 10 to 13 years were not significantly different, but from the age of 14 to 19 years, the mean NC of males was significantly higher than that of the females. This is consistent with similar studies in children and adolescents in the United States of America (1) and Turkey (8) and may be explained by the fact that male sex hormones (androgens) are associated with deposition of fat in the upper body, of which the neck region is a part of (6). Female sex hormones on the other hand are associated with an increase in lower body fat which includes the thighs and gluteal region (6). Also, pubertal changes in boys, marked by the appearance of secondary sexual characteristics, are usually as a result of increased androgenic secretion from the gonads which begin to be seen at about 11 to 12 years of age (23). These androgens also cause laryngeal and pharyngeal enlargement in males (24). As the androgenic secretions continue to increase in the latter adolescent years, it is not surprising that its effect on the neck was evident in the increasing neck circumference of the male subjects in this study, throughout their mid- and late adolescent years.

BMI was found to significantly correlate positively with NC, as was seen in other studies (1, 8). The fact that NC was significantly different in the two BMI categories studied in both genders (normal and high BMI) indicates that it would do well as marker for overweight and obesity.

This study proposed NC cutoff values for overweight and obesity per period of adolescence, and not per singular age group, as were seen in similar studies carried out in areas of higher overweight/obesity prevalence

(1, 8). This may be useful in places with relatively low prevalence of overweight and obesity so that larger numbers of overweight or obese people are available to evaluate optimal cutoff values, as opposed to the fewer numbers or none that may be available when evaluated per singular age. Secondly, the larger groupings per adolescent period means that fewer cutoff values need to be remembered by a busy clinician who may not have time to refer to a chart which would be a necessity if the cutoff values were provided per singular age group.

ROC analysis routinely provides predictive values for the diagnostic test being evaluated, being NC in this instance. The positive predictive values of NC were low, while the negative predictive values were high. These values depend on disease prevalence and are not unwavering characteristics of the diagnostic test that is being evaluated (25). Hence, they could be misleading in an area of relatively low prevalence such as Nigeria. A more clinically useful measure is the Likelihood Ratio which is independent of prevalence (25).

With the high sensitivities and less remarkable specificities of the proposed NC cutoff values, along with their high positive likelihood ratios and low negative likelihood ratios, NC can serve as a good screening tool for overweight and obesity in Nigerian adolescents. Further evaluation of those with a positive test based on the NC value can then be carried out with more specific tests of overweight and obesity.

A limitation of this study is that its findings may not be extended to adolescents outside the school community like those already employed or in other institutions of learning.

CONCLUSION

This study has demonstrated that neck circumference is a useful screening tool for obese and overweight adolescents. It is simple and cost effective and so envisaged to be beneficial in primary health care settings. Hopefully this picks-up potential candidates for the two morbidities and avert the more sinister associated complications.

ACKNOWLEDGMENTS

The authors will like to thank all the students that participated in this research, their parents and the volunteer measurers. Special thanks also go to certain individuals who supported this research financially namely Air Vice Marshall Nicholas Spiff (Rtd), Air Commodore Simon Okwuokei (Rtd) and Air Commodore Adebayo Bolajoko (Rtd).

The authors declare that they have no conflict of interest. Informed consent was obtained from the parent/guardian of each participant involved in this study. Assent was obtained from each participant. This study was conducted in accordance with the 1964 Declaration of Helsinki and its subsequent amendments.

REFERENCES

[1] Nafiu OO, Burke C, Lee J, Voepel-Lewis T, Mabiya S, Tremper KK. Neck circumference as a screening measure for identifying children with high body mass index. Pediatrics 2010;126:306-10.

[2] Akinpelu AO, Oyewole OO, Oritogun KS. Overweight and obesity: Does it occur in Nigerian adolescents in an urban community? Int J Biomed Hlth Sci 2008;4:11-7.

[3] Owa JA, Adejuyigbe O. Fat Mass, fat mass percentage, body mass index and MUAC in a healthy population of Nigerian children. J Trop Pediatr 1997;43:13–9.

[4] Alton I. The overweight adolescent In: Stang J, Story M, eds. Guidelines for adolescent nutrition services, 1st ed. Minneapolis, MN: Centre for Leadership, Education and Training in Maternal and Child Nutrition, Division of Epidemiology and Community health, School of Public health, University of Minnesota,2005:77-91.

[5] Centers for Disease Control and Prevention. Overweight and obesity, 2010. URL: htpp/www/cdc.gov/obesity/defining.html.)

[6] Kissebah AH, Krakower GR. Regional adiposity and morbidity. Physiol Rev 1994;74:761-811.

[7] Ben-Noun L, Sohar E, Laor A. Neck circumference as a simple screening measure for identifying overweight and obesity patients. Obes Res 2001;9:470–4.

[8] Hatipoglu N, Mazicioglu MM, Kurtoglu F, Kenderci M. Neck Circumference: An additional tool for screening overweight and obesity in childhood. Eur J Pediatr 2010;169:733-9.

[9] Ministry of Science and Technology, 2011. URL: http/www/lagosstate.gov.ng.)

[10] Marfell-Jones M, Olds T, Stewart A, Carter JEL, eds. International standards for anthropometric assessment. Underdale, SA: International Society for the Advancement of Kinanthropometry (ISAK), 2001.

[11] Center for Disease Control and Prevention. Children's BMI tool for schools. Assessing your weight, 2011. URL: http://www.cdc.gov/healthyweight/assessing/bmi/childrens_bmi/tool_for_schools.html.)

[12] Bewick V, Cheek L, ball J. Statistics review 13: Receiver operating characteristic curves. Crit Care 2004;8:508-12.

[13] Wang Y, Lobstein T. Worldwide trends in childhood overweight and obesity. Int J Pediatr Obes 2006;1:11-25.

[14] Dietz WH. Health consequences of Obesity in youth: Childhood predictors of adult disease. Pediatrics 1998;101:S18–S25.

[15] Reilly JJ, Wilson D. The ABC of obesity: Childhood obesity. BMJ 2006;333:1207–10.

[16] Deurenberg P, Deurenberg-Yap M. Validation of skinfold thickness and handheld impedance measurements for estimation of body fat percentage among Singaporean Chinese, malay and Indian subjects. Asia Pacific J Clin Nutr 2002;11:1-7

[17] Lean MJ, Han TS. Waist worries. Am J Clin Nutr 2002;76:699–700.

[18] Hall TMB, Cole TJ. What use is the BMI? Arch Dis Child 2006;91:283-6

[19] Dehgan M, Merchant AT. Is bioelectrical impedance accurate for use in large epidemiological studies? Nutr J 2008;7:26-33.

[20] Horlick M, Hediger ML. Measurement matters. J Pediatr 2010;156:178.

[21] Sjostrom CD, Hakangard AC, Lissner L, Sjostrom L. Body compartment and subcutaneous adipose tissue distribution-risk factor patterns in obese subjects. Obes Res 1995;3:9–22.

[22] Laberge RC, Vaccani JP, Gow RM, Gaboury I, Hoey L, Katz SL. Inter- and intra-rater reliability of neck circumference measurements in children. Pediatr Pulm 2009;44:64–9.

[23] Heird WC. Nutrition. In: Kleigman RM, Behrman RE, Jenson HB, Stanton BF, eds. Nelson textbook of pediatrics, 18th ed. Philadelphia, PA: Saunders Elsevier, 2007:209-14.

[24] Marcell AV. Adolescence. In: Kliegman RM, Behrman RE, Jenson HB, Stanton BF, eds. Nelson textbook of pediatrics, 18th ed. Philadelphia, PA: Saunders Elsevier, 2007:60-5.

[25] Sedighi I. Interpretation of diagnostic tests: Likelihood ratio; vs predictive value. Iran J Pediatr 2013;23:717.

In: Nigeria: Perspectives of Health
Editors: Ariel Tenenbaum et al.
ISBN: 978-1-53618-090-9

Chapter 14

SERUM TRIGLYCERIDE-TO-HIGH-DENSITY LIPOPROTEIN CHOLESTEROL RATIO: PROFILE AND ITS USE AS SURROGATE FOR INSULIN RESISTANCE PREVALENCE IN OVERWEIGHT/OBESE ADOLESCENTS

Alphonsus N Onyiriuka[1,*], MBBS, FMCPaed,
Nosakhare J Iduoriyekemwen[2], MBBS, FWACP(Paed)
and Wilson E Sadoh[3], MBBS, FWACP(Paed)

[1]Endocrinology and Metabolism Unit
[2]Nephrology and [3]Cardiology Units,
Department of Child Health,
University of Benin Teaching Hospital,
Benin City, Nigeria

* Corresponding Author's Email: alpndiony@yahoo.com.

Abstract

Triglyceride-to-high-density lipoprotein cholesterol (TG/HDL-C) ratio is a cost-effective tool to predict and identify insulin resistance and cardiometabolic risk in overweight/obese children and adolescents. The present study described the pattern and distribution of TG/HDL-C ratio as well as its use in determining the prevalence of insulin resistance in overweight/obese adolescents. *Methods:* In this school-based cross-sectional study, the serum lipid levels (total cholesterol (TC), high density lipoprotein cholesterol (HDL-C), triglyceride (TG), and low density lipoprotein cholesterol (LDL-C) of overweight/obese and normal weight adolescents were measured The TG/HDL-C ratio was calculated for subjects and controls. Insulin resistance was defined by serum TG/HDL-C ratio greater than 2.27. *Results:* In the overweight/obese participants, 53.1% and 38.8% were in middle and upper tertiles of TG/HDL-C concentration ratios, respectively. The mean TG/HDL-C ratios was higher in overweight/obese than normal weight participants; 1.92 ± 0.64 (95% CI = 1.74-2.10) versus 1.68 ± 0.31 (95% CI = 1.59-1.77); p-value < 0.05. The prevalence of insulin resistance as defined by TG/HDL-C > 2.27 was significantly higher in overweight/obese than normal weight adolescents; 35.4% (95% CI = 28.6-42.2) versus 12.2% (95% CI = 7.5-16.9); Odds ratio (OR) = 4.0. *Conclusion:* Clinicians can apply TG/HDL-C ratio to the standard lipid screening in order to identify overweight/obese adolescents with increased risk of insulin resistance and cardiometabolic disorders.

Introduction

The triglyceride-to-high-density lipoprotein cholesterol (TG/HDL-C) ratio reflects the association between triglyceride (TG) and high density lipoprotein cholesterol (HDL-C), depicting the balance between atherogenic and protective lipoproteins (1). TG/HDL-C ratio has a good correlation with LDL particle size in children and adolescents (2). This lipid ratio has been found to be a useful marker in detection of early functional and morphological vascular changes as well as nonalcoholic fatty liver disease (NAFLD) in paediatric population (3, 4). The results of some studies indicate that elevated TG/HDL-C ratio in children and adolescents is associated with increased risk of insulin resistance, high blood pressure, metabolic syndrome and NAFLD (4-7). In a study in China, it was concluded that TG/HDL-C ratio has a discriminatory power in detecting potential metabolic syndrome in the paediatric age group (8). In the same study, the authors stated in their conclusion that TG/HDL-C ratio was a better index than homeostasis model assessment insulin resistance (HOMA-IR) for screening for metabolic syndrome in obese children and adolescents. Urbina et al. (9) demonstrated that elevated TG/HDL-C ratio was an independent determinant of arterial stiffness in adolescents and young adults, suggesting that the use of TG/HDL-C ratio may also be helpful in identifying young adults requiring intervention to prevent arteriosclerotic cardiovascular disease. In a study involving Spanish children, aged 2-17 years, it was demonstrated that TG/HDL-C ratio > 2 is an effective and relatively cheap biomarker to identify the early stage of potential metabolic syndrome in overweight/obese paediatric population at any age and pubertal status (10). Therefore, some researcher have recommended that TG/HDL-C ratio should be routinely determined from traditional serum lipid levels to assess atherogeneity of dyslipidaemias which is critical for prevention of cardiometabolic diseases (4, 5).

The results of several studies have demonstrated that TG/HDL-C ratio is a useful surrogate for insulin resistance in the paediatric age group (3, 6, 11, 12). The interest in TG/HDL-C ratio as a tool for estimating insulin resistance was because of ease of measurement in routine clinical settings and cost-effectiveness. Within this context, other components of insulin sensitivity indices such as insulin, C-peptide, leptin, cytokines and free fatty acids are more expensive to measure. In resource-limited countries, simple affordable screening tool is an attractive option. There are lines of evidence showing that TG/HDL-C ratio is a relatively simple cost-effective way to identify apparently healthy insulin-resistance children and adolescents with increased cardiometabolic risk (5, 13). Various cutoff points of serum TG/HDL-C ratio have been used as a surrogate in different studies to define insulin resistance in children and adolescents. In this regard, Pacifico et al. (4) used ≥1.98 and Hannon et al. [15] used ≥ 3.0 as definitions, respectively. In two separate studies, serum TG/HDL-C ratio greater than 2.27 was used in identifying overweight/obese children and adolescents with insulin resistance (7, 14). The results of a study in Malaysian children, aged 9 to 16 years, revealed that children with insulin resistance had a significantly higher TG/HDL-C ratio than those without insulin resistance (16). In the same report, the authors stated that the odds of having insulin resistance was about 2.5 times higher for those in the upper tertile of TG/HDL-C ratio compared with those in the two lower tertiles. Di Bonito et al. (5) demonstrated that TG/HDL-C ratio $\geq$ 2.0 is associated with several cardiometabolic risk factors and preclinical signs of cardiac abnormalities in a group of Caucasian children and adolescents, suggesting that this lipid ratio may also predict insulin-resistance-mediated organ damage. Inter-ethnic differences in muscle, liver and abdominal fat partitioning has been demonstrated, suggesting that the degree of insulin resistance may be different for the same body mass index, depending on ethnicity (17, 18). It has been reported that TG/HDL-C ratio $\geq$ 2.2 was significantly associated with impaired glucose tolerance (IGT) in children and adolescents, reflecting its usefulness in identifying overweight/obese individuals at risk of IGT (19) and future type 2 diabetes (20, 21). To the best of our knowledge, there is no published report on the pattern, distribution and use of TG/HDL-C ratio as a surrogate for identifying insulin resistance in overweight/obese Nigerian children and adolescents. The aim of the present study is to describe the pattern and distribution of TG/HDL-C ratio as well as its use in determining the prevalence of insulin resistance in overweight/obese adolescents.

OUR STUDY

This was a school-based cross-sectional study involving an urban secondary school in Egor Local Government Area (LGA) of Edo State, Nigeria. The study was conducted over one-month period, 1st to 30th June, 2016. Ethical clearance certificate was obtained from Research and Ethics Committee of the College of Medical Sciences, University of Benin, Benin City. The administrative head of the school and the ministry of education gave permission for the conduct of the study. Written informed consent was obtained from the parent(s)/caregiver of each of the study subjects. We obtained verbal accent from each of the participants and emphasized to them that their participation was entirely voluntary.

Study group and sampling technique

In this study, the first secondary school in a list of alphabetically arranged private secondary schools in Egor LGA was selected. The list of private secondary schools was obtained from the Edo State Ministry of Education (22). Thereafter, students within the age group of 10-16 years were randomly selected. Each of the selected students was given a written note explaining the nature of the study as well as a questionnaire to be completed by their parent(s). The subjects (high BMI, $\geq 85^{th}$ percentile) and controls (normal BMI, 5th to $< 85^{th}$ percentile) were matched for age and gender. The socio-economic status and ethnicity of the subjects and controls were largely similar. Excluded from the study were students with positive history or obvious clinical evidence of hypothyroidism, liver disease, chronic kidney disease, Cushing syndrome, diabetes mellitus or who are on drugs such as corticosteroids or oral contraceptives.

Anthropometric measurements

Following a standard procedure (23) the height was measured to the nearest 0.1 cm, using a Holtian portable anthropometer and the weight was measured to the nearest 0.1 kg, using a Seca Scale Balance with the subject in light clothing and bare foot. If a duplicate measurement differed by > 0.5 cm or > 0.5 kg respectively, a third measurement was performed and the average of the two closest measurements was recorded as the final value. To eliminate inter-observer error, all the anthropometric measurements were performed by one of the authors. The body mass index of each of the subjects was computed, using the standard formula (23). The blood pressure of the participants was measured by one of the authors and steps were taken to minimize errors.

Blood sample collection and serum lipid profile analysis

Venous blood sample was collected after the details of the intended procedure was explained to the participants. The participants maintained their usual dietary pattern within the past three days preceding the study. Following an overnight fast (at least 12-hour fast), 5ml of venous blood was collected into appropriate sample container without anticoagulant and stored at 8^0C. After one hour, all samples were centrifuged at 3000rpm for 15 minutes and the serum aliquots were stored at -20^0C until assayed. The serum concentrations of total cholesterol (TC), high-density lipoprotein-cholesterol (HDL-C) and triglycerides (TG) and low-density lipoprotein-cholesterol (LDL-C) were determined, using automated analyzer with commercially available kits and following strictly the manufacturer's instructions throughout the assay procedures.

Definitions

TG/HDL-C ratio was calculated as TG(mg/dl) divided by HDL-C (mg/dl). The participants were grouped into tertiles based on their serum TG/HDL-C concentration ratios as follows: lower tertile < 1.2; middle tertile 1.2 to < 2.0; and upper tertile ≥ 2.0 (6). Participants with TG/HDL-C ratio in the upper tertile were considered as having high TG/HDL-C ratio (5, 6). Serum TG/HDL-C ratio greater than 2.27 defined insulin resistance (7, 14). High serum triglyceride concentrations was defined as triglyceride $\geq$ 130mg/dl (for children $\geq$10 years old) and low HDL-C concentration as $<$ 40mg/dl, according the criteria proposed by National Heart, Lung and Blood Institute (NHLBI) in 2011 (24). Normal weight, overweight and obesity were defined as BMI between 5th to $< 85^{th}$, 85th to $< 95^{th}$ and $\geq 95^{th}$ percentiles, respectively.

Statistical analysis

The data were collated and entered into an Excel spread sheet. Accuracy of the data entered was double checked. Subsequently, data were analysed, using Microsoft Excel and SPSS (Statistical Package for Social Sciences) version 20.0. The descriptive statistics reported are mean, standard deviation, confidence intervals, tertiles and percentages. Differences between means were tested with t-test and proportions were tested using Z-test. Significant p-values were set at < 0.05.

FINDINGS

A total of 98 (49 subjects and 49 controls) students were investigated. There were 29 girls and 20 boys in each of the two groups. The mean age of the participants was 12.1 ± 1.2 years. The characteristics of subjects and controls are displayed in Table 1. Overweight/obese participants had a significantly higher mean BMI and waist circumference.

As shown in Table 2, 38.8% of overweight/obese participants were in the upper tertiles of TG/HDL-C concentration ratio. The mean TG/HDL-C ratio was higher in overweight/obese than in normal weight adolescents; 1.92 ± 0.64 (95% Confidence Interval, CI = 1.74-2.10) versus 1.68 ± 0.31 (95% CI = 1.59-1.77); t-statistic 2.362, $p < 0.05$. Table 3 shows that the prevalence of insulin resistance (TG/HDL-C ratio > 2.27) was 35.4% (95% CI = 28.6-42.2) and 12.2% (95% CI = 7.5-16.9) in overweight/obese and normal weight adolescents, respectively; Odds ratio (OR) = 4.0. When TG/HDL-C ratio ≥ 3.0 was applied as cutoff point for insulin resistance, only two (4.1%) overweight/obese but none in normal weight group demonstrated insulin resistance. In both overweight/obese and normal weight groups none had serum triglyceride level equal or greater than 130 mg/dl.

Table 1. Characteristics of the subjects (overweight/obese) and controls (normal weight) according to gender

Characteristics	Subjects Male	Controls Male	t-statistic (p-value)	Subjects Female	Controls Female	t-statistic (p-value)
Mean weight (kg)	52.3 ± 6.4	39.1 ± 7.8	9.158 (< 0.001)	40.6 ± 5.2	36.3 ± 8.4	3.047 (< 0.01)
Mean height (cm)	149.3 ± 6.8	142.4 ± 6.6	5.097 (< 0.01)	146.8 ± 7.3	140.3 ± 5.6	4.945 (< 0.01)
Mean BMI(kg/m^2)	27.32. ± 72	16.8 ± 2.15	9.800 (< 0.001)	28.7 ± 3.3	17.5 ± 3.50	16.300 (< 0.001)
Mean WC (cm)	83.2 ± 4.9	68.8 ± 4.1	15.777 (< 0.001)	88.9 ± 5.2	69.1 ± 6.7	16.342 (< 0.001)
Mean HC (cm)	90.3 ± 10.6	70.8 ± 8.8	9.908 (< 0.001)	102.3 ± 8.7	72.5 ± 8.6	17.052 (< 0.001)
Mean WC/HC ratio	0.90 ± 0.08	0.85 ± 0.05	3.710 (< 0.001)	0.86 ± 0.05	0.80 ± 0.06	5.378 (< 0.001)
Mean SBP (mmHg)	107.3 ± 10.2	103.5 ± 9.9	1.871 (> 0.05)	105.0 ± 9.4	101.5 ± 9.3	1.853 (> 0.05)
Mean DBP(mmHg)	70.0 ± 6.7	63.6 ± 8.8	4.051 (< 0.001)	65.7 ± 9.1	62.1 ± 9.6	1.905 (> 0.05)
Mean TC (mg/dl)	136.3 ± 26.6	124.2 ± 23.8	1.652 (> 0.05)	141.0 ± 25.8	133.2 ± 20.9	1.243 (> 0.05)
Mean HDL-C(mg/dl)	37.0 ± 5.2	37.2 ± 4.6	0.132 (> 0.05)	38.1 ± 6.1	37.1 ± 5.3	0.655 (> 0.05)
Mean TG (mg/dl)	101.8 ± 27.2	90.3 ± 25.6	1.414 (>0.05)	102.5 ± 23.7	95.5 ± 22.7	1.129 (> 0.05)
Mean LDL-C(mg/dl)	68.5 ± 24.2	65.7 ± 25.8	0.363 (> 0.05)	76.7 ± 20.2	73.1 ± 18.8	0.690 (> 0.05)

WC = Waist circumference; HC = Hip circumference; SBP = Systolic blood pressure; DBP = Diastolic blood pressure.

Table 2. Frequency of tertiles of TG/HDL-C concentration ratios in overweight/obese and normal weight subjects

Tertiles of TG/HDL-C Ratio	Normal weight (n = 49) No (%)	Overweight/obese (n = 49) No (%)	Z-statistic (p-value)
Lower (< 1.2)	9(18.4)	4(8.2)	1.504(>0.05)
Middle (1.2 to < 2.0)	23(46.9)	26(53.1)	0.615(>0.05)
Upper (≥ 2.0)	17(34.7)	19(38.8)	0.421(>0.05)

TG = Triglyceride; HDL-C = High density lipoprotein cholesterol.

Table 3. Prevalence of insulin resistance in overweight/obese and normal weight participants based on TG/HDL-C ratio greater than 2.27

Category of participant	Prevalence of insulin resistance (TG/HDL-C ratio > 2.27) Number Percent	Z-statistic (p-value)
Normal weight (n = 49)	6 12.2	
Overweight/obese (n = 49)	17 35.4	2.802(<0.01)
Total (N = 98)	23 23.5	

TG = Triglyceride; HDL-C = High density lipoprotein cholesterol.

DISCUSSION

Nearly every four out of ten of our overweight/obese adolescents demonstrated upper tertile TG/HDL-C concentration ratios (≥2.0) which is considered elevated. Other investigators have reported a similar finding (6). Considering the report of Di Bonito et al. (5), this finding is worrisome. Di Bonito et al. (5) demonstrated that TG/HDL-C ratio ≥ 2.0 is associated with increased risk of cardiometabolic disorders in a group of Caucasian children and adolescents. In the same study, they found an association with preclinical signs of cardiac abnormalities. The public health implication is that TG/HDL-C ratio in upper tertile constitutes a non-communicable healthcare burden because it may also predict insulin-resistance-mediated organ damage (5). In addition, some studies have shown that an elevated TG/HDL-C ratio (≥2.0) identified the onset of metabolic alterations related to metabolic syndrome (MetS), such as decreased insulin sensitivity and altered lipid profile (5, 10, 25). The elevated TG/HDL-C ratio found in the present study was mainly due to low serum HDL-C concentrations as none of the participants, in both subjects and controls, had serum triglyceride level in the abnormal range (i.e., ≥ 130 mg/dl in individuals ≥10 years old), using the criteria proposed by National Heart, Lung and Blood Institute (NHLBI) in 2011 (24). The public health implication is that specific dietary modification capable of increasing serum HDL-C level is indicated in our adolescent population.

As in other reports (6), the mean TG/HDL-C concentration ratio was statistically significantly higher in overweight/obese than normal weight adolescents in this study. Further confirming that overweight/obesity is a risk factor for abnormal TG/HDL-C ratio in adolescents.

We found a 4-fold greater odd of elevated TG/HDL-C ratio (>2.27) for overweight/obese than normal weight adolescents. In the present study, as in others (7, 14), TG/HDL-C ratio greater than 2.27 was considered a surrogate for insulin resistance. Based on this criteria, prevalence of insulin resistance was statistically significantly higher in overweight/obese than in normal weight group. Our finding is in consonance with previous reports (6, 13, 19). Adolescents with such abnormal lipid ratio profile are at increased risk of exhibiting impaired glucose tolerance and may develop type 2 diabetes in future (20, 21). It has been documented that when insulin sensitivity is impaired, compensatory hyperinsulinaemia is produced. Over time, pancreatic beta cell dysfunction occurs, promoting development of type 2 diabetes (25). Within this context, TG/HDL-C ratio is a useful clinical tool for identifying adolescents at risk of MetS and low insulin sensitivity (5, 26). Some pathophysiologic mechanisms have been proposed to explain the link between obesity and insulin resistance. Obesity results in proinflammatory state, starting in metabolic cells (adipocyte, hepatocyte, or myocyte). This is followed by recruitment of macrophages with subsequent release of inflammatory cytokines that predispose toward insulin resistance (27). Chen et al. (28) have demonstrated that musclin, a novel skeletal muscle-derived secretory factor has a strong relationship with obesity-associated insulin resistance. A higher ratio of TG/HDL-C implies a poor health status not only because the amount of fat in circulation is larger but also because the amount of healthy cholesterol in circulation is lower. Cardiometabolic risk factors tend to precede the development of atherosclerosis in obese children and adolescents (29). Therefore, lifestyle modification is required in adolescents with TG/HDL- C concentration ratio > 2.27. When a higher cutoff point of TG/HDL-C ratio of ≥ 3.0 was applied, the frequency of insulin resistance was nearly 9 times lower in overweight/obese adolescents, suggesting that TG/HDL-C ratio > 2.27 was a more appropriate cutoff point in the paediatric age group.

Strengths and weaknesses of the study

The strength of the study is that the subjects and controls were derived from a single well defined source population. In addition, matching increased the statistical precision of estimates, thereby allowing smaller sample size. The weakness of the study was that the study population was derived from a single school, making it possible that the sample was not representative of adolescents in the source population. Despite this limitation, it provided baseline epidemiological data (the first among Nigerian adolescents) on the subject and could serve as an initial point for future study.

CONCLUSION

In conclusion, clinicians can apply TG/HDL-C ratio to the standard lipid screening in order to identify overweight/obese adolescents with increased risk of insulin resistance and cardiometabolic disorders.

ACKNOWLEDGMENTS

We have no conflict of interest in this study.

REFERENCES

[1] Millián J, Pintó X, Muñoz A, Zúñiga M, Rubiés-Prat J, Pallardo LF, Musana L, et al. Lipoprotein ratios: physiological significance and clinical usefulness in cardiovascular prevention. Vasc Health Risk Manag 2009;5:757-65.

[2] Maruyama C, Imamura K, Teramoto T. Assessment of LDL particle size by triglyceride/HDL-cholesterol ratio in non-diabetic, healthy subjects without prominent hyperlipidemia. J Atheroscler Thromb 2003;10:186-91.

[3] McLaughlin T, Reaven G, Abbasi F, Lambendola C, Saad M, Water J, Simon J, Krauss RM. Is there a simple way to identify insulin-resistant individuals at increased risk of cardiovascular disease? Am J Cardiol 2005;96:399-404.

[4] Pacifico L, Bonci E, Andreoli G, Romaggioli S, Di Miscio R, Lombardo C, Chiesa C. Association of serum triglyceride-to-HDL cholesterol ratio with carotid artery intima thickness, insulin resistance and nonalcoholic fatty liver disease in children and adolescents. Nutr Metab Cardiovasc Dis 2014;24:737-43.

[5] Di Bonito P, Moio N, Scilla C, Cavuto L, Sibilio G, Sanguigno E, et al. Usefulness of the high triglyceride-to-HDL-cholesterol ratio to identify cardiometabolic risk factors and preclinical signs of organ damage in outpatient children. Diabetes Care 2012;35:158-62.

[6] Yoo DY, Kang YS, Kwon EB, Yoo EG. The triglyceride to high density lipoprotein cholesterol ratio in overweight Korean children and adolescents. Ann Pediatr Endocrinol Metab 2017;22:158-63.

[7] Üstyol A, Kökali F, Duru NS, Elevli M. Association of serum triglyceride –to-high-density lipoprotein cholesterol ratio with insulin resistance and nonalcoholic fatty liver disease in children and adolescents. Med Bull Haseki 2017;55:286-91.

[8] Liang J, Fu J, Jiang Y, Dong G, Wang X, Wu W. Triglyceride and high-density lipoprotein-cholesterol ratio compared with homeostasis model assessment insulin resistance indexes in screening for metabolic syndrome in Chinese obese children: a cross sectional study. BMC Pediatr 2015;15:138-44.

[9] Urbina EM, Khoury PR, McCoy CE, Dolan LM, Daniels SR, Kimball TR. Triglyceride to HDL-C ratio and increased arterial stiffness in children, adolescents and adults. Pediatrics 2013;131:e1082-92.

[10] Caurtero BG, Vergaz AG, Lacalle CG, Escudero VS, Salado LS, de Larramendi CH. Leptin and cytokines are not the best markers of metabolic syndrome. Horm Res Paediatr 2018;90(Suppl 1):P2-P128.

[11] Salazar MR, Carbajal HA, Espeche WG, Dulbecco CA, Aizpuua M, Marillet AG, Echeverria RF, Reaven GM. Relationships among insulin resistance, obesity, diagnosis of the metabolic syndrome and cardiometabolic risk. Diabetes Vasc Dis Res 2011;8:109-16.

[12] Kim-Dorner SJ, Deuster PA, Zeno SA, Remaley AT, Poth M. Should triglycerides and the triglyceride to high-density lipoprotein cholesterol ratio be used as surrogates for insulin resistance? Metabolism 2010;59:299-304.

[13] Oliveira AC, Oliveira AM, Oliveira N, Oliveira A, Almeidia M, Veneza LM, Oliveira AL, Adan L, Ladeia AM. Is triglyceride to high density lipoprotein cholesterol ratio a surrogate for insulin resistance? Health 2013;5:481-5.

[14] Giannini C, Santoro N, Caprio S, Kim G, Lartaud D, Shaw M, Pierpont B, Weiss R. The triglyceride-to-HDL cholesterol ratio: association with insulin resistance in obese youths of different ethnic backgrounds. Diabetes Care 2011;34:1869-74.

[15] Hannon TS, Basha F, Lee SJ, Janosky J, Arslantan SA. Use of markers of dyslipidemia to identify overweight youth with insulin resistance. Pediatr Diabetes 2006;7:260-6.

[16] Zati Iwan NAK, Jalatudin MY, Mohl Zin RMW, Fuziah MZ, Hua Hong JY, Abqaryah Y, Mokhtar AH, Wan Nazaimoon WM. Triglyceride to high density lipoprotein cholesterol ratio is associated with insulin resistance in overweight and obese children. Sci Rep 2017;7:40055. doi:10.1038/srep 40055(2017).

[17] Liska D, Dufour S, Zern TL, TaksalI MS, Cali AM, et al. Interethnic differences in muscle, liver and abdominal fat partitioning in obese adolescents. PLoS One 2007;2:e5690.

[18] Weiss R, Nassar H, Sinnreich R, Kark JD. Differences in the triglyceride to high density lipoprotein cholesterol ratio between Palestinian and Israeli adults. PLoS One 2015;10(1):e0116617.

[19] Manco M, Grugni G, Di Pietro M, Balsamo A, Di Candia S, Morino GS, et al. Triglyceride-to-HDL-cholesterol ratio as a screening tool for impaired glucose tolerance in obese children and adolescents. Acta Diabetol 2016;53:493-8.

[20] He S, Wang S, Chen X, Jiang L, Peng Y, Li L, Wan L, Cui K. Higher ratio of triglyceride to high density lipoprotein cholesterol may predispose to diabetes mellitus: 15-year prospective study in a general population. Metab Clin Exp 2012;61:30-6.

[21] Copeland KC, Zeiter P, Geffner M, Gaundalini C, Higgins J, Hirst K, Kaufman FR, Linder B. Characteristics of adolescents and youth with recent onset type 2 diabetes:the TODAY cohort at baseline. J Clin Endocrinol Metab 2011;96:159-67.

[22] Ministry of Education, Benin City. Department of Planning, Research and Statistics. Directory of pre-primary, primary, junior and senior secondary institutions in Edo State. Benin City: Ministry of Education, 2006.

[23] Marfell-Jones M, Olds T, Stew A, Carter L. International standards for anthropometric assessment. Melbourne: International Society for the Advancement of Kinanthropometry, 2006.

[24] Expert Panel on Integrated Guidelines for Cardiovascular Health and Risk Reduction in Children and Adolescents; summary report. Expert panel on integrated guidelines for cardiovascular health and risk reduction in children and adolescents; National Heart, Lung and Blood Institute. Pediatrics 2011;128(Suppl 5):S213-56.

[25] Pineda CA. Metabolic syndrome: definition and history criteria. Colomb Med 2008;39:96-106.

[26] Baez-Duarte BG, Zamora-Ginez I, González-Duarte R, Torres-Rasgado E, Ruiz-Vivanco G, Pérez-Fuentes R, The Multidisciplinary Research Group of Diabetes. Triglyceride/high-density lipoprotein cholesterol (TG/HDL-C) index in a reference criterion of risk for metabolic syndrome (MetS) and low insulin sensitivity in apparently healthy subjects. Gac Med Mex 2017;153:152-8.

[27] van den Berg E, Bissseli GJ, Stehouwer CDA, Kapptle LJ, Heine RJ, et al. Ten-year time course of risk factors for increased carotid intima-media thickness: the Hoorn Study. Eur J Cardiovasc Prev Rehabil 2010;17:168-74.

[28] Chen WJ, Liu Y,Sui YB, Yang HT, Chang HR, Tang CS, Qi YF, Zhang J, Yin XH. Positive association between musculin and insulin resistance in obesity: evidence of a human study and animal experiment. Nutr Metab 2017;14:46-57.

[29] Greenberg AS, Obin MS. Obesity and the role of adipose tissue in inflammation and metabolism. Am J Clin Nutr 2006;83(Suppl 1):461S-5.

In: Nigeria: Perspectives of Health
Editors: Ariel Tenenbaum et al.
ISBN: 978-1-53618-090-9

Chapter 15

PSEUDOHYPOPARATHYROIDISM: A RARE CAUSE OF HYPOCALCAEMIA

Alphonsus N Onyiriuka**, MBBS, FMCPaed and Victor A Esedume, MBBS

Endocrinology and Metabolism Unit, Department of Child Health, University of Benin Teaching Hospital, Benin City, Nigeria

ABSTRACT

Pesudohypoparathyroidism (PHP) is a rare heterogeneous group of disorders due to genetic defects in the hormone receptor adenylate cyclase system and whose common feature is end-organ unresponsiveness to parathyroid hormone. In all its forms, it is biochemically characterized by hypocalcaemia, hyperphosphataemia and elevated level of serum parathyroid hormone. In this report, we present a case of a 15-year-old Nigerian boy who had symptoms of both acute and chronic hypocalcaemia. He was referred to our hospital because of chest pain. Prior to his referral, he has had an episode of generalized tonic-clonic seizure. Further inquiry revealed history of muscle cramps and pain in the bones and joints. Anthropometric measurements revealed that

* Corresponding Author's Email: alpndiony@yahoo.com.

weight, height and body mass index were all below the 5th percentile for age and gender. Trousseau's sign was positive in the patient. The laboratory findings include hypocalcaemia (serum calcium 0.18 mmol/L), hyperphosphataemia (serum phosphate 11.2 mmol/L), elevated parathyroid hormone (serum parathyroid hormone 7.8 pmol/L) level and normal serum magnesium (serum magnesium 0.72 mmol/L) level. Results of both the renal and thyroid function tests were normal. The diagnosis of PHP was delayed probably because of the rarity and heterogeneity of this clinical entity. Conclusion: Pseudohy poparathyroidism should be considered in any child or adolescent with persistent hypocalcaemia in the presence of elevated serum parathyroid hormone level, particularly if renal function tests and serum magnesium level are normal.

INTRODUCTION

Pesudohypoparathyroidism (PHP) is a rare heterogeneous group of disorders whose common feature is end-organ unresponsiveness to parathyroid hormone due to receptor or post-receptor defect (1). In all its forms, it is biochemically characterized by hypocalcaemia, hyperphosphataemia and elevated serum parathyroid hormone (PTH) level (1). The classification of PHP is based on the phenotype and cellular cyclic adenosine monophosphate (cAMP) response to exogenous parathyroid hormone administration. Phenotypically, some patients have the constellation of features of Albright Hereditary Osteodystrophy (AHO) which includes short stature, obesity, round face, shortened metacarpals and metatarsals and multiple hormonal resistances (1). PHP is divided into two major groups, types I and II based on renal response to exogenous PTH administration (1). Type I PHP is further subdivided into types Ia, Ib, Ic (1). In patients with PHP types Ia and Ic features of AHO and multiple hormonal resistance are present. In contrast, patients with PHP types Ib and type II features of AHO and multiple hormonal resistance are absent (1). Very recently, the EuroPHP Network proposed a novel nomenclature/classification from PHP to "inactivating PTH/PTHrP signalling disorder (iPPSD)" (2). According to EuroPHP Network, the merits of the new terminology include (i) defines the common mechanism responsible for all diseases (ii) does not require a confirmed genetic defect (iii) avoids ambiguous terms like 'pseudo' and (iv) eliminates the clinical or molecular overlap between diseases. The authors concluded that the use of this nomenclature and classification will facilitate the development of rationale and comprehensive international guidelines for the diagnosis and treatment of iPPSDs (2).

The prevalence of PHP is largely unknown. The reported prevalence rates are 3.4 and 11 per million population in Japan and Denmark, respectively (3, 4). An extensive search of the literature did not reveal any report on the subject from Nigeria. Thus, emphasizing the rare nature of this clinical entity.

A CASE STORY

A 15-year-old Nigerian boy referred to the Endocrinology and Metabolism unit, University of Benin Teaching Hospital (UBTH), because of persistent symptomatic hypocalcaemia despite treatment with oral calcium and vitamin D3. The patient was referred to UBTH from a private hospital because of recurrent chest pain of two years duration. The chest pain was sharp and retrostenal. In addition, he has recurrent muscle cramps, bone and joint pain which are aggravated by strenuous exercise and writing. In the past one month, the frequency of the muscle cramps, bone and joint pain has increased (coupled with the persistent hypocalcaemia) warranting referral to a paediatric endocrinologist. There is no history of disturbances of taste, smell, vision or hearing. Developmental milestones including pubertal development appear normal. He had an episode of seizure (probably hypocalcaemic) three years ago and no repeats since then. There was no history suggestive of chronic kidney or liver disease. The index patient is the second of three children (all boys) in the family. No family history of similar symptoms. He had an average academic performance. Physical examination revealed an apparently healthy-looking boy with weight 35.5 kg (<5th percentile), height 147 cm (<5th percentile) and body mass index 16.4 kgm^{-2} (<5th percentile). He had a positive Trousseau's sign and no shortening of metacarpals or metatarsals. He has no evidence of dental anomaly or subcutaneous calcification or cataract or moniliasis. His blood pressure was 80/60 mmHg. Examination of the body systems was unremarkable. The results of laboratory investigations showed that serum urea, electrolytes, creatinine as well as urinalysis were all normal. The results of his thyroid function tests were normal. Echocardiogram did not reveal any structural anomaly of the heart. His haemoglobin phenotype is AS. The initial laboratory findings are summarized in Table 1.

Table 1. Summary of initial biochemical results initial

Parameter	Results	Comments
Serum total calcium	0.18 mmol/L	Very low
Serum corrected calcium	0.13 mmol/L	Very low
Serum phosphate	11.2 mmol/L	Very high
Parathyroid hormone	7.8 pmol/L	High
Serum magnesium	0.72 mmol/L	Within normal limits
Serum albumin	4.2 g/L	Within normal limits
Serum alkaline phosphatase	411 µU/L	Within normal limits
24-hour-urine calcium	1.92 mmol/24hrs	Low
Random blood glucose	5.1 mmo/L	Within normal limits

Table 2. Serial serum calcium and phosphate concentrations

Serial no	Serum total calcium mmol/L	Comments	Serum phosphate mmol/L	Comments
Test 1	0.93	Very low	1.87	High
Test 2	1.33	Low	2.00	High
Test 3	1.70	Low	2.84	Very high
Test 4	1.93	Low	2.13	High
Test 5	1.13	Very low	2.62	Very high
Test 6	1.86	Low	2.17	High

He had correction of the symptomatic hypocalcaemia using intravenous 10% calcium gluconate, followed by maintenance oral calcium but the hypocalcaemia persisted as shown in Table 2. In addition, his serum phosphate levels remained high.

We considered a clinical diagnosis of pseudohypoparathyroidism. Based on this diagnosis, we planned further laboratory investigation. In this regard, the Parathyroid Hormone Response Test with assay of urinary phosphate and cyclic adenosine monophosphate (cAMP) was planned. We were unable to perform this investigation because of inadequate laboratory facility in our hospital and financial constraint prevented using commercial medical laboratories outside. Oral calcium supplement was continued and the vitamin D was changed to oral 1 α-vitamin D (calcitriol).

DISCUSSION

In the index case, the presence of hypocalcaemia, hyperphosphataemia, elevated level of serum parathyroid hormone and normal serum magnesium level without evidence of underlying systemic disorder, such as chronic kidney disease suggested a diagnosis of pseudohypoparathyroidism. In addition, the absence of the phenotypic features of Albright Hereditary Osteodystrophy suggests a subtype diagnosis of PHP type Ib or type II (1). The clinical manifestations in our patient included an episode of seizure and recurrent episodes of muscle cramps, pain in the chest, bone and joints. The single episode of seizure may be related to severe hypocalcaemia at that time. His hypocalcaemic condition may have become clinically evident following the pubertal growth spurt, which is known to be associated with a relatively higher calcium requirements (5). This clinical scenario in our patient is not surprising as Kabicek et al. (6) reported two cases of PHP in two adolescent boys; one with low back pain and the other with seizure. Although vitamin D deficiency with biochemical findings resembling PHP types I and II has been described (7), alone it is unlikely to cause significant hypocalcaemia as observed in our patient without a rise in alkaline phosphatase level. Our patient's serum alkaline phosphatase level was normal, thereby negating the diagnosis of vitamin D deficiency.

The etiologic diagnosis of the persistent hypocalcaemia was delayed for 2 to 3 years in our patient despite several medical consultations. This is not surprising as similar observation has been reported from Italy (5) and India (9). In the case reported from India, the patient had symptoms of chronic hypocalcaemia for 10 years before diagnosis (9). The difficulty in diagnosing PHP is due to its rarity as well as the varying phenotypic aspects. The clinical implication is that full biochemical investigation of calcium-phosphate metabolism is required in any child or adolescent with signs and symptoms of hypocalcaemia to avoid missed aetiologic diagnosis. In this regard, it is imperative to always measure serum levels of calcium, phosphate, magnesium and parathyroid hormone. In addition, assessment of the renal function is required to exclude hyperphosphataemia secondary to chronic kidney disease (10). Measurement of serum magnesium is important because low serum magnesium is known to impair both the secretion and function of parathyroid hormone (1).

We encountered some challenges in evaluation and management of the index case. Inadequate laboratory facility prevented us from performing the Parathyroid Hormone Response Test with assay of urinary phosphate and cAMP to distinguish between PHP types I and II and molecular studies (demonstration of the mutated G-protein) to confirm our diagnosis of PHP. The parents of the patient were experiencing difficulties procuring oral calcitriol, which is the preferred form of vitamin D for therapy. Despite this limitation, we are reasonably certain that the patient has PHP (with either types Ib or II being the likely subtype). It is possible that in future, if the novel classification proposed by EuroPHP Network (2) is adopted, more appropriate diagnosis could be achieved with less sophisticated laboratory investigations, particularly in resource-limited countries with inadequate laboratory facilities.

CONCLUSION

In conclusion, the learning point is that full biochemical investigation of calcium-phosphate metabolism is required in any child or adolescent with signs and symptoms of hypocalcaemia to avoid missed aetiological diagnosis. Pseudohypoparathyroidism should be considered in any child or adolescent with persistent hypocalcaemia associated with elevated parathyroid hormone level, particularly if serum magnesium level and renal function are normal.

REFERENCES

[1] Roth KS, Ward RJ, Chan JCM, Sarafoglou K. Disorders of calcium, phosphate and bone metabolism. In: Sarafoglou K, ed. Pediatric endocrinology and inborn errors of metabolism. New York: McGraw Hill, 2009:619-68.

[2] Thiele S, Mantovani G, Barlier A, Boldrin V, Bordoogna P, De Sanctis L, et al. From pseudohypoparathyroidism to inactivating PTH/PTHrP signalling disorder (iPPSD), a novel classification proposed by the EuroPHP network. Eur J Endocrinol 2016;125(6):P1-17.

[3] Nakamura Y, Matsumoto T, Tamakoshi A, Kawamura T, Seino Y, Kasuga M, Yanagawa H, Ohno Y. Prevalence of idiopathic hypoparathyroidism and pseudohypoparathyroidism in Japan. J Epidemiol 2000;10:29-33.

[4] Underbjerg L, Sikjaer T, Mosekilde L, Rejnmark L. Pseudohypoparathyroidism – epidemiology, mortality and risk of complications. Clin Endocrinol (Oxf) 2016;84:904-11.

[5] Mesias M, Seiquer I, Navarro MP. Calcium nutrition in adolescence. Crit Rev Food Sci Nutr 2011;51(3):195-209.

[6] Kabicek P, Katilek S, Bayer M, St?pán JJ. Two cases of pseudohypoparathyroidism in adolescent boys. Acta Univ Carol Med (Praha) 1994;40(1-4):53-6.

[7] Seki T, Yamamoto M, Kimura H, Tsuiki M, Ono M, Miki N, Takano K, Sato K. Vitamin D deficiency in two young adults with biochemical findings resembling pseudohypoparathyroidism type I and type II. Endocr J 2010;57:715-44.

[8] Donghi V, Mora S, Zamproni I, Chiumello G, Weber G. Pseudohypoparathyroidism, an often delayed diagnosis: a case series. Cases Journal 2009;2:6734-8.

[9] Dosi KV, Ambaliyu AP, Joshi HK, Patell RD. Pseudohypoparathyroidism, rare cause of hypocalcaemia. J Clin Diagnostic Res 2013;7(10):2288-9.

[10] Wesseling K, Bakkaloglu S, Salusky I. Chronic kidney disease mineral and bone disorder in children. Pediatr Nephrol 2008;23:195-207.

SECTION TWO: ACKNOWLEDGMENTS

In: Nigeria: Perspectives of Health
Editors: Ariel Tenenbaum et al.
ISBN: 978-1-53618-090-9

Chapter 16

ABOUT THE EDITORS

Ariel Tenenbaum, MD is the director of the Center for Children with Chronic Diseases at the Hadassah-Hebrew University Medical Center at the Mount Scopus Campus, Jerusalem, Israel. He graduated the Hadassah-Hebrew University Medical School and after pediatric residency at the Department of Pediatrics at Mount Scopus Campus, he continued his work at the hospital as a senior pediatric consultant and teacher of medical students. In 2004 he was appointed the head of the new Israeli Down syndrome program in the hospital. In 2005 he started the pre-adoption clinic together with Professor Isaiah D. Wexler. In 2012 he opened the Hadassah Intellectual and Developmental Disability Multidisciplinary Evaluation Center in collaboration with the Ministry of Social Affairs. He co-founded the Disability Studies Center at the Hebrew University, where he teaches students from humanities and social studies. He was recently appointed as a child development consultant. In 2019 he was elected to the Israeli Pediatric Association Committee and serves as its scientific secretary. His main research topics are disabilities, adoption, chronic diseases and general pediatrics. He has published numerous book chapters, edited several books, and published dozens of scientific articles in international journals. Email: tene@hadassah.org.il

Kehinde K Kanmodi, BDS, Dip. FM, PGDPM, PGDE, PGDPSCR, CPMP, ACIPM, AISQEM is a dental surgeon, lecturer, multidisciplinary researcher, and manager affiliated with Cephas Health Research Initiative Inc, Ibadan (head office), Community Health Officers' Training Programme, Usmanu Danfodiyo University Teaching Hospital, Sokoto, National Teachers' Institute, Department of Political Science of the National Open University of Nigeria, Abuja, Nigerian Institute of Management, Abuja, Chartered Institute of Project Management, Lagos, and Dental Clinic, Kebbi Medical Centre, Kalgo, Nigeria. He is the founder, chair of the board of trustees and executive director of the Cephas Health Research Initiative Inc – a not-for-profit nongovernmental, non-partisan and indigenous health research organization in Nigeria. He has over 80 publications to his credit. He is also a peer reviewer to ten journals in the field of health and medical sciences. He plans to have his PhDs in Health Promotion and Socio-behavioral Sciences, and International Development. Email: kehindekanmodi@gmail.com

Joav Merrick, MD, MMedSci, DMSc, born and educated in Denmark is professor of pediatrics, Division of Pediatrics, Hadassah Hebrew University Medical Center, Mt Scopus Campus, Jerusalem, Israel and Kentucky Children's Hospital, University of Kentucky, Lexington, Kentucky United States and professor of public health at the Center for Healthy Development, School of Public Health, Georgia State University, Atlanta, United States, the former medical director of the Health Services, Division for Intellectual and Developmental Disabilities, Ministry of Social Affairs and Social Services, Jerusalem, the founder and director of the National Institute of Child Health and Human Development in Israel. Numerous publications in the field of pediatrics, child health and human development, rehabilitation, intellectual disability, disability, health, welfare, abuse, advocacy, quality of life and prevention. Received the Peter Sabroe Child Award for outstanding work on behalf of Danish Children in 1985 and the International LEGO-Prize ("The Children's Nobel Prize") for an extraordinary contribution towards improvement in child welfare and well-being in 1987. In 2017 appointed a Kentucky Colonel by the

Commonwealth of Kentucky, the highest honor the governor can bestow to a person. Email: jmerrick@zahav.net.il

In: Nigeria: Perspectives of Health
Editors: Ariel Tenenbaum et al.
ISBN: 978-1-53618-090-9

Chapter 17

About the Center for Children with Chronic Diseases and Down Syndrome Center Jerusalem, Israel, Department of Pediatrics, Mt Scopus Campus, Hadassah Hebrew University Medical Center, Jerusalem, Israel

Chronic illnesses are common among children. These conditions last longer than a year and require continuous medical care and special needs. It is estimated that 10-20% of children in developed countries have one or more chronic condition. Advances in medicine and technology lead to an increase in the survival rate and longevity of children with chronic diseases and special needs. The severity of different chronic illnesses is variable, but there are many similarities. The child with a chronic illness faces physical, social, and emotional challenges. Therefore, medical care is not sufficient without rehabilitative service and emotional care for the child and his family.

Chronic illnesses are time and energy consuming. These children go through treatments, procedures and many healthcare visits. At home they often continue treatments as well, e.g., physiotherapy, breathing support machines and medications. This lifestyle may have detrimental effect on the child's social and emotional well-being, and similarly affect his parents and siblings.

CENTER FOR CHILDREN WITH CHRONIC DISEASES

The aim of the Center for Children with Chronic Diseases at the Hadassah-Hebrew University Medical Center at the Mount Scopus Campus, Jerusalem, is to enhance medical care, comfort and well-being of patients and their families in the hospital and beyond. The center provides integrated and comprehensive care for these patients. This includes extensive support services and helping their families cope with the burden of care.

Numerous pediatric specialty programs and medical divisions have been established in the center to care for specific chronic conditions; among them are cystic fibrosis, Down syndrome, diabetes mellitus, familial dysautonomia, neuromuscular diseases, rheumatic diseases, feeding disorders and metabolic diseases. All these programs include evaluation and support from common services in the center: Nursing, nutrition, psycho-social care, speech therapy, physiotherapy and more.

The center works as a "one stop shop" for these children; As many services as possible, under one roof, on the same visit. Centralizing the care enables parents to come to one location to receive care. The physicians and nurses coordinate the care of the children thereby alleviating some of the burden of care off the families.

Children who are included in the programs of the center usually need returning visits to various medical specialists, consultations by multidisciplinary health professionals and performing diagnostic tests e.g., blood work, x-rays and respiratory functions. Some children may need hospitalization or palliative care. The center can concentrate all diagnostic and follow-up testing, medical surveillance and treatment in the hands of an experienced staff who knows the child and his unique situation.

The center is situated close to the entrance of the hospital and the families can access it without going through the main hospital building. In the center there are ten rooms for consultations. In addition, there are dedicated rooms for tests, e.g., respiratory functions, blood tests, sweat test and more. There is a large space with eight beds for continuous treatments, for example intravenous immunoglobulins and biological medications. In this space several unique tests are performed as well, for example growth hormone test and allergy challenge tests. There is also a special room for procedures, in which children can go through painful treatments with appropriate anesthetics and surveillance.

A special classroom in the center is operated by the ministry of education. In the classroom, children can continue their studies or play and interact with other children, in arts and crafts and many other programs.

The center is surrounded by a large healing garden that is partially maintained by the children themselves.

Conclusion

In conclusion, we believe that the "all inclusive" model of a center for children with chronic conditions is beneficial for the children and their families in terms of health and quality of life, and that this model is currently the best service for them.

Contact

Ariel Tenenbaum, MD, Isaiah D Wexler, MD, PhD
Center for Children with Chronic Diseases, Department of Pediatrics,
Mt Scopus Campus, Hadassah Hebrew University Medical Center,
Jerusalem, Israel
Email: TENE@hadassah.org.il

In: Nigeria: Perspectives of Health
Editors: Ariel Tenenbaum et al.
ISBN: 978-1-53618-090-9

Chapter 18

About the Cephas Health Research Initiative Inc in Nigeria

The Cephas Health Research Initiativ (CHRI) Inc in Nigeria was established in 2016 as a not-for-profit, non-partisan, non-government organization to help improve the health and wellbeing of the people of Nigeria.

Mission

The mission of CHRI Inc is to improve the health and wellbeing of Nigerians through health education, advocacy and health research that informs policy makers.

Vision

To become a leading health and development non-governmental organization in Africa

Humanitarian services

The CHRI Inc is well known for her humanitarian services in the Nigeria society. Since 2016, the organization has been able to launch several laudable health research and health education programs including the Campaign for Head and Neck Cancer Education (CHANCE) Program, Child Health And Wellbeing (CHAW) Program, and Fight Pain (FP) Program (of which the Sakkiya Project is a subset). From these programs, thousands of individuals have been surveyed, while hundreds have been educated on health matters. From the surveys carried out by this organization, multiples of book chapters and articles have been published as peer reviewed scientific documents. The findings made from their surveys are also forwarded to the concerned ministries of health in Nigeria as a guide for policy makers.

Collaborators

The CHRI Inc has multidisciplinary collaborators from all the geopolitical zones in Nigeria. Also, some collaborators are outside Nigeria. The organization welcomes hands that are interested in collaboration.

Contact

Kehinde Kanmodi, BDS, Dip. FM, PGDPM, PGDE, PGDPSCR, ACIPM, AISQEM
Chair, Board of Trustees, and Executive Director
Cephas Health Research Initiative Inc, Ibadan, Nigeria.
Email: kanmodikehinde@yahoo.com, kehindekanmodi@gmail.com

In: Nigeria: Perspectives of Health
Editors: Ariel Tenenbaum et al.
ISBN: 978-1-53618-090-9

Chapter 19

About the National Institute of Child Health and Human Development in Israel

The National Institute of Child Health and Human Development (NICHD) in Israel was established in 1998 as a virtual institute under the auspices of the Medical Director, Ministry of Social Affairs and Social Services in order to function as the research arm for the Office of the Medical Director. In 1998 the National Council for Child Health and Pediatrics, Ministry of Health and in 1999 the Director General and Deputy Director General of the Ministry of Health endorsed the establishment of the NICHD.

Mission

The mission of a National Institute for Child Health and Human Development in Israel is to provide an academic focal point for the scholarly interdisciplinary study of child life, health, public health, welfare, disability, rehabilitation, intellectual disability and related aspects of human development. This mission includes research, teaching, clinical work, information and public service activities in the field of child health and human development.

Service and academic activities

Over the years many activities became focused in the south of Israel due to collaboration with various professionals at the Faculty of Health Sciences (FOHS) at the Ben Gurion University of the Negev (BGU). Since 2000 an affiliation with the Zusman Child Development Center at the Pediatric Division of Soroka University Medical Center has resulted in collaboration around the establishment of the Down Syndrome Clinic at that center. In 2002 a full course on "Disability" was established at the Recanati School for Allied Professions in the Community, FOHS, BGU and in 2005 collaboration was started with the Primary Care Unit of the faculty and disability became part of the master of public health course on "Children and society". In the academic year 2005-2006 a one semester course on "Aging with disability" was started as part of the master of science program in gerontology in our collaboration with the Center for Multidisciplinary Research in Aging. In 2010 collaborations with the Division of Pediatrics, Hadassah Hebrew University Medical Center, Jerusalem, Israel around the National Down Syndrome Center and teaching students and residents about intellectual and developmental disabilities as part of their training at this campus.

Research activities

The affiliated staff have over the years published work from projects and research activities in this national and international collaboration. In the year 2000 the International Journal of Adolescent Medicine and Health and in 2005 the International Journal on Disability and Human Development of De Gruyter Publishing House (Berlin and New York) were affiliated with the National Institute of Child Health and Human Development. From

2008 also the International Journal of Child Health and Human Development (Nova Science, New York), the International Journal of Child and Adolescent Health (Nova Science) and the Journal of Pain Management (Nova Science) affiliated and from 2009 the International Public Health Journal (Nova Science) and Journal of Alternative Medicine Research (Nova Science). All peer-reviewed international journals.

National collaborations

Nationally the NICHD works in collaboration with the Faculty of Health Sciences, Ben Gurion University of the Negev; Department of Physical Therapy, Sackler School of Medicine, Tel Aviv University; Autism Center, Assaf HaRofeh Medical Center; National Rett and PKU Centers at Chaim Sheba Medical Center, Tel HaShomer; Department of Physiotherapy, Haifa University; Department of Education, Bar Ilan University, Ramat Gan, Faculty of Social Sciences and Health Sciences; College of Judea and Samaria in Ariel and in 2011 affiliation with Center for Pediatric Chronic Diseases and National Center for Down Syndrome, Department of Pediatrics, Hadassah Hebrew University Medical Center, Mount Scopus Campus, Jerusalem.

International collaborations

Internationally with the Department of Disability and Human Development, College of Applied Health Sciences, University of Illinois at Chicago; Strong Center for Developmental Disabilities, Golisano Children's Hospital at Strong, University of Rochester School of Medicine and Dentistry, New York; Centre on Intellectual Disabilities, University of Albany, New York; Centre for Chronic Disease Prevention and Control, Health Canada, Ottawa; Chandler Medical Center and Children's Hospital, Kentucky Children's Hospital, Section of Adolescent Medicine, University of Kentucky, Lexington; Chronic Disease Prevention and Control Research

Center, Baylor College of Medicine, Houston, Texas; Division of Neuroscience, Department of Psychiatry, Columbia University, New York; Institute for the Study of Disadvantage and Disability, Atlanta; Center for Autism and Related Disorders, Department Psychiatry, Children's Hospital Boston, Boston; Department of Pediatric and Adolescent Medicine, Western Michigan University Homer Stryker MD School of Medicine, Kalamazoo, Michigan, United States; Department of Paediatrics, Child Health and Adolescent Medicine, Children's Hospital at Westmead, Westmead, Australia; International Centre for the Study of Occupational and Mental Health, Düsseldorf, Germany; Centre for Advanced Studies in Nursing, Department of General Practice and Primary Care, University of Aberdeen, Aberdeen, United Kingdom; Quality of Life Research Center, Copenhagen, Denmark; Nordic School of Public Health, Gottenburg, Sweden, Scandinavian Institute of Quality of Working Life, Oslo, Norway; The Department of Applied Social Sciences (APSS) of The Hong Kong Polytechnic University Hong Kong.

Targets

Our focus is on research, international collaborations, clinical work, teaching and policy in health, disability and human development and to establish the NICHD as a permanent institute in Israel in order to conduct model research.

Contact

Professor Joav Merrick, MD, MMedSci, DMSc
National Institute of Child Health and Human Development, Jerusalem, Israel.
Email: jmerrick@zahav.net.il

SECTION THREE: INDEX

Index

D

E

F

G

H

I

J

K

L

M

N

O

P